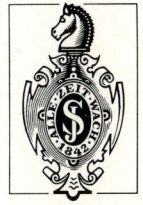

Heinz-Dieter Neumann

Introduction to Manual Medicine

Translated and Edited by Wolfgang G. Gilliar

Foreword by Philip E. Greenman

With 62 Figures

Springer-Verlag Berlin Heidelberg New York
London Paris Tokyo Hong Kong

Heinz-Dieter Neumann, M.D.
Orthopedic Surgeon
(Past President of FIMM)
Bühlertalstraße 45
FRG-7580 Bühl/Baden

Wolfgang G. Gilliar, D.O.
National Rehabilitation Hospital
102 Irving Street NW
USA-Washington, D.C. 20010-2949

Translation of the 3rd German edition:
Manuelle Medizin
© Springer-Verlag Berlin Heidelberg 1983, 1986, 1989

ISBN 3-540-50612-8 Springer-Verlag Berlin Heidelberg New York
ISBN 0-387-50612-8 Springer-Verlag New York Berlin Heidelberg

Library of Congress Cataloging-in-Publication Data
Neumann, Heinz-Dieter. [Manuelle Medizin. English] Introduction to manual medicine /
Heinz-Dieter Neumann ; translated and edited by Wolfgang G. Gilliar ; foreword by Philip
E. Greemann. p. cm. Translation of: Manuelle Medizin. Bibliography: p. Includes index.
ISBN 0-387-50612-8 (U.S.: alk. paper)
1. Manipulation (Therapeutics) I. Gilliar, Wolfgang G. II. Title. [DNLM: 1. Manipulation,
Orthopedic. 2. Physical Medicine. WB 535 N492m]
RM724.N4813   1989   615.8'2-dc20   DNLM/DLC   89-6309

This work is subject to copyright. All rights are reserved, whether the whole or part of the
material is concerned, specifically the rights of translation, reprinting, reuse of illustrations,
recitation, broadcasting, reproduction on microfilms or in other ways, and storage in data
banks. Duplication of this publication or parts thereof is only permitted under the
provisions of the German Copyright Law of September 9, 1965, in its version of June 24,
1985, and a copyright fee must always be paid. Violations fall under the prosecution act of
the German Copyright Law.

© Springer-Verlag Berlin Heidelberg 1989
Printed in Germany

The use of general descriptive names, registered names, trademarks, etc. in the publication
does not imply, even in the absence of a specific statement, that such names are exempt
from the relevant protective laws and regulations and therefore free for general use.

Product Liability: The publisher can give no guarantee for information about drug dosage
and application thereof contained in this book. In every individual case the respective user
must check its accuracy by consulting other pharmaceutical literature.

Typesetting, printing and binding: Appl, Wemding
2119/3145-543210 - Printed on acid-free paper

Foreword

This volume is a welcome contribution to the literature on manual medicine. It is concise and accessible, yet covers the field comprehensively. It presents a synthesis of the past current literature and provides a valuable overview. Dr. Neumann, for many years a student, practitioner, teacher, and now international leader in this field, demonstrates his deep understanding of the diverse theories and vocabularies current in many schools of manual medicine, and presents the various viewpoints and approaches in an easily readable fashion.

This book is of assistance to the neophyte student as well as the experienced practitioner. From the basics of palpation to the clinical cases, both typical and complex, the reader's knowledge is enhanced with each succeeding page.

Introduction to Manual Medicine represents a valuable addition to the library of all practitioners treating patients with musculoskeletal problems.

April 1989, East Lansing, Michigan   Philip E. Greenman,
                                            D.O., F.A.A.O.

Preface

When I was working as a resident orthopedist at the University Hospital in Tübingen, Germany, I saw a patient in the orthopedic clinic who complained of headaches. This patient, who apparently had previously seen a practitioner of manual medicine, stated that his atlas must have "popped out of place" and asked me to "fix it, to put it back in place." Despite my having had extensive orthopedic training up to that time, I did not unterstand what the patient actually meant, and could not help him further.

I discussed this particular case with my chief, Professor Dr. Hans Mau, who advised me to familiarize myself with the field of manual medicine. So I started out by taking the various courses offered, read the literature available at that time (admittedly rather limited), and traveled extensively to meet with other colleagues practicing manual medicine.

In 1971 I began teaching manual medicine courses at one of the two schools in Germany. Through my involvement as president of the German Association of Manual Medicine and the International Federation of Manual Medicine I was able to make many useful international contacts and gain an overview of both the differences and similarities in practices in the various coutries and their societies.

This book, then, is the result of all these experiences. It was written with two purposes in mind. The first is to give a basic overview of the present day practice and scope of the field of manual medicine. If, in addition, the information thus provided helps reduce certain existing prejudices towards this field, I will be delighted. With the information presented here, the reader should be able to make his own judgement.

The second purpose is to provide background material for basic courses in manual medicine, both practical and theoretical, which is how the German editions have been used in the Federal Republic of Germany and Austria.

I would like to thank all of my friends throughout the world for their information, instruction and advice. For the English edition, which is largely based on the third German edition, I would like to thank Professors Myron C. Beal and Philip E. Greenman, both of Michigan State University, College of Osteopathic Medicine. I appreciate their support and critical advise. My special thanks go to Dr. Wolfgang G. Gilliar, who, with great diligence and interest in the subject matter, not only translated the original German text but helped in incorporating new material known in the English-speaking community.

Again, I would like to thank Springer-Verlag for their continued support and cooperation.

Bühl, July 1989   Heinz-Dieter Neumann

Table of Contents

1	**Manual Medicine - A Historical Review**	1
2	**Fundamentals of Manual Medicine**	3
2.1	Somatic Dysfunction	3
2.1.1	Definition	4
2.1.2	Hypotheses for Somatic Dysfunction	4
2.2	Manual Medicine - A Theoretical Model	5
2.2.1	Mechanical Circuit	6
2.2.2	Nervous System and Reflex Circuit	7
2.2.3	Practical Applications	10
2.2.4	Diagnostic Signs of Somatic Dysfunction	12
2.2.5	Causes of a Somatic Dysfunction	13
3	**Diagnosis in Manual Medicine**	14
3.1	General Evaluation	15
3.2	General Manual Medicine Diagnosis (the Screen, Gross Manual Examination).	16
3.2.1	Surface Orientation	16
3.2.2	Layer Palpation	19
3.3	Specific Examination by Manual Medicine Techniques (the Scan)	22
3.3.1	Biomechanical Considerations	22
3.4	The Segmental Manual Medicine Examination	34
3.4.1	Palpatory Assessment of Joint Mobility (Motion Testing)	38
3.4.2	Palpatory Assessment of Localized Segmental Irritation	46
3.4.3	Palpatory Assessment of Peripheral Segmental Irritation	52
3.5	X-Ray Examination of the Spine	53
3.5.1	Radiographic Technique	54
3.5.2	Normal Radiographic Findings	56
3.6	Examination of Extremity Joints	57

4 Manual Therapy 62

4.1 Soft Tissue Techniques 64
4.2 Mobilization Techniques Without Impulse 65
4.2.1 Passive Mobilization 65
4.2.2 Active Mobilization 68
4.3 Indirect Techniques 71
4.3.1 Functional Techniques 71
4.3.2 Strain-Counterstrain Technique (After Jones) 73
4.4 Low Amplitude, High Velocity Thrust Technique
(Mobilization with Impulse) 73
4.5 Other Techniques 76
4.5.1 Myofascial Technique 76
4.5.2 Cranio-Sacral Technique 76
4.6 Reevaluation 76

5 Contraindications to Manual Medicine 78

5.1 Inflammatory Processes 78
5.2 Destructive Processes 79
5.3 Trauma with Associated Anatomical Changes 79
5.4 Osteoporosis 79
5.5 Degenerative Changes 80
5.6 Vertebral Artery 81
5.7 Psychological Disturbances 84

6 Hypermobility 85

6.1 General Hypermobility 85
6.2 Local Pathological Hypermobility 86

7 Cases from Clinical Practice 88

7.1 Cervical Syndrome 88
7.1.1 Upper Cervical Syndrome 88
7.1.2 Lower Cervical Syndrom 91
7.2 Thoracic Syndrome 92
7.3 Lumbar Syndrome 94
7.4 Sciatica 96
7.4.1 Differential Diagnosis of Lumbar Disc Herniation . . . 96
7.4.2 Sacro-iliac Joints 97
7.4.3 Coccydynia 100
7.5 Extremity Joints 100

8	**Afterword**	102
9	**References**	103
10	**Subject Index**	107

1 Manual Medicine – A Historical Review

"Bone setting" is probably as old as mankind itself. Many earlier cultures seem to have produced their own experts who, by the use of their hands, effect treatment so as to alleviate discomfort associated with the spine and extremity joints. From my own childhood in Silesia, for instance, I recall some shepherds who were considered to be masters in the application of manipulation (here, manipulation is a more general term denoting any therapeutic procedure in which the hands are used to both diagnose a musculoskeletal problem and treat the patient).

Manual medicine can be dated to the time of Hippocrates (460–377 B.C.) who was the first occidental physician to describe the techniques of manipulation in his treatise "Peri Arthron." Unfortunately, with the fall of the Roman Empire much of the medical knowledge from these times was lost. Some of the knowledge can be found in other cultures, for instance in the writings of Islamic scholars, such as Avicenna, 980–1037 A.D. Until more recently, however, the medical and surgical writings in Europe made little mention of manipulative therapy.

Not unlike other fields of medicine, manipulative therapy can trace its roots to folklore practices. Similar to the modern practitioner of internal medicine, who expanded on the knowledge of herbal lore, or the present day surgeon whose predecessor is the barber, today's practitioners of manual medicine find their roots in the bone setters. In contrast to the traditional fields of medicine, manipulative therapy has been met more with skepticism than with acceptance by the medical community. Perhaps scientific progress with its astounding advances in pharmacological and surgical modalities in the nineteenth and twentieth centuries is to some extent responsible for the fact that manual medicine has been more or less ignored by the traditional schools of medicine.

During the past 30 to 40 years, however, manual medicine not only has become more popular but, in the hands of scientifically oriented physicians, has made significant progress especially in investigating and elucidating some of the underlying mechanisms responsible for the success of manipulation. Manual medicine has been strongly influenced by osteopathic medicine and chiropractic.

In 1874, Andrew Taylor Still, M.D., proposed a new philosophy of the healing arts, which he termed "Osteopathy." In 1894, he founded the first school of osteopathy in Kirksville, Missouri, where successful candidates were awarded the degree of "Doctor of Osteopathy." Still, who may have been influenced by immigrant bone setters in the Midwest, had taken the art of healing by means of manipulation of the spine and extremity joints and developed it into a teachable science. Even though strongly dealing with and emphasizing the structural importance of the spine and extremities, the field of osteopathic medicine includes surgery, obstetrics and the use of medications. The osteopathic profession today has 15 accredited colleges, some of which are affiliated with state universities. After completing four years of premedical training and four years of medical school training, the graduate of an osteopathic school (D.O.) is granted the same privileges as his allopathic counterpart (M.D.). Every osteopathic graduate has received, in addition to the regular medical curriculum, a minimum 400 hours of instruction and practice in structural diagnosis and treatment of the spine and extremity joints. The medically trained osteopaths (D.O.) are not to be mixed up with lay "osteopaths" working in Great Britain and France (Paterson and Burn 1985).

The founder of chiropractic was Daniel David Palmer, a Canadian-American grocer, who, in 1895, founded the School of Chiropractic in Davenport, Iowa. The practice of chiropractic consists primarily of the diagnosis of disturbances of the musculoskeletal system (i.e. the so called "subluxation") and the non-invasive treatment of reversible dysfunctions ("adjustments") but has expanded to include nutritional counseling and the use of vitamins, etc. In recent years, the chiropractic profession has engaged in scientific investigation of the phenomena related to the use of manipulation.

In 1966 the North American Academy of Manipulative Medicine was established by a group of allopathic physicians, including Godfrey, Mennell, Rubin, Rudd and Travell. Since 1977, osteopathic physicians have become members of this association which most recently changed its name to the North American Academy of Musculoskeletal Medicine (NAAMM). The objective of the Academy is to advance the field of manual medicine and offer educational opportunities for physicians.

The North American Academy of Musculoskeletal Medicine is a member of FIMM, the International Federation of Manual Medicine, which was founded in 1968 and presently represents 21 countries.

A similar development took place in other English speaking countries, such as Great Britain, Australia, and New Zealand, and also in nearly all West European countries.

2 Fundamentals of Manual Medicine

Manual medicine concerns itself with the physiology, pathophysiology and prevention of reversible functional disturbances affecting the musculoskeletal system. The practice of manual medicine comprises those diagnostic and therapeutic techniques that aid in the localization and remedy of functional disorders associated with the spine and the extremity joints.

2.1 Somatic Dysfunction

Reversible functional disorders of the joints may express themselves as either decreased or increased mobility. In this book, dysfunctions associated with increased mobility are discussed at a later point, in the chapter entitled "Hypermobility" (p. 85).

In the coming chapters we will concentrate on dysfunctions that result in decreased joint movement. Several terms have been used in various countries to describe this entity of altered or impaired function of related body components of the somatic system (body framework). In this text, we use the term "somatic dysfunction," which has been registered in the United States in the ICD-9-CM (International Classification of Disease) replacing the antiquated term "osteopathic lesion." According to the Glossary of Osteopathic Terminology (Ward 1981), this entity includes associated changes in the skeletal, arthrodial, and myofascial structures, and related vascular, lymphatic, and neural elements. In other countries, the term "segmental and peripheral articular dysfunction" has been used, whereas in Europe, in particular in the German-speaking countries, the rather mechanical term "blockage" has become a standard term. In this book, in order to ensure consistency, the term "somatic dysfunction" has been used wherever applicable.

2.1.1 Definition

> Somatic dysfunction with motion restriction may be defined as and result in:
> (a) The presence of a reversible dysfunction expressed as decreased mobility; this impaired movement may be seen at any point along the physiological range of motion in a joint (from neutral to the limit of the joint's anatomical range). The restriction may be in one or several directions and joint play is usually decreased as well.
> (b) Muscles that are associated with the incriminated joint(s) usually being contracted in a particular pattern.
> (c) Possible further effects on the function of tissues and internal organs that are segmentally related to the restricted joint.
>
> *The presence of a somatic dysfunction is the only indication for manual therapy!*

2.1.2 Hypotheses for Somatic Dysfunction

Numerous theories and hypothetical postulates have been proposed concerning the etiology of a somatic dysfunction. The following list is but a limited representation of the major etiologies suggested by various authors:

- dysfunction in the circulation of tissue fluid (Still 1908),
- subluxation[1] (Palmer 1933),
- nerve impingement (Palmer 1933),
- meniscus compression (Zukschwerdt et al. 1960; Dörr 1962),
- derangement of intervertebral discs (Maigne 1963; Cyriax 1969; Fisk 1977),
- impaired gliding (translatory movement) of joint surfaces,
- dysfunction arising from changes in the reflexive neural regulation associated with disturbances in a joint (Korr 1975; Dvořák and Dvořák 1983).

There are, of course, many more hypothetical postulates which attempt to explain the possible causes of somatic dysfunctions. It is most likely insufficient to seek an explanation for a dysfunction in one particular body system, that is to interpret a somatic dysfunction as being only of articulatory, circulatory, muscular or neuroreflexive origin. The joint, intervertebral disc, muscles and nervous system all may be viewed as imbedded in more global feedback mechanisms, so called "circuits," that interrelate the entire organism. A somatic dysfunction is presumed to be due to an aberration in any one or more of these feedback circuit components.

---

[1] The term "subluxation" should no longer be used in connection with or as a substitute for the entity called somatic dysfunction, as it has been a major source of misunderstanding in traditional medicine. This term denotes either an incomplete dislocation or a restriction of motion of a joint in a position exceeding normal physiological motion, although the anatomical limits have not been exceeded (Glossary of Osteopathic Terminology).

2.2 Manual Medicine – A Theoretical Model

In this section, we shall use the apophyseal (facet) joint as an example of our present theoretical understanding of the causes, clinical symptomatology and significance of a somatic dysfunction. Essentially, the same principles hold true for a peripheral joint as well, where, however, mechanical factors seem to be the rule rather than a neuroreflexive problem.

For this discussion, the apophyseal joint is considered part of two regulatory circuits, the mechanical circuit and the neuroreflexive circuit (Fig. 1).

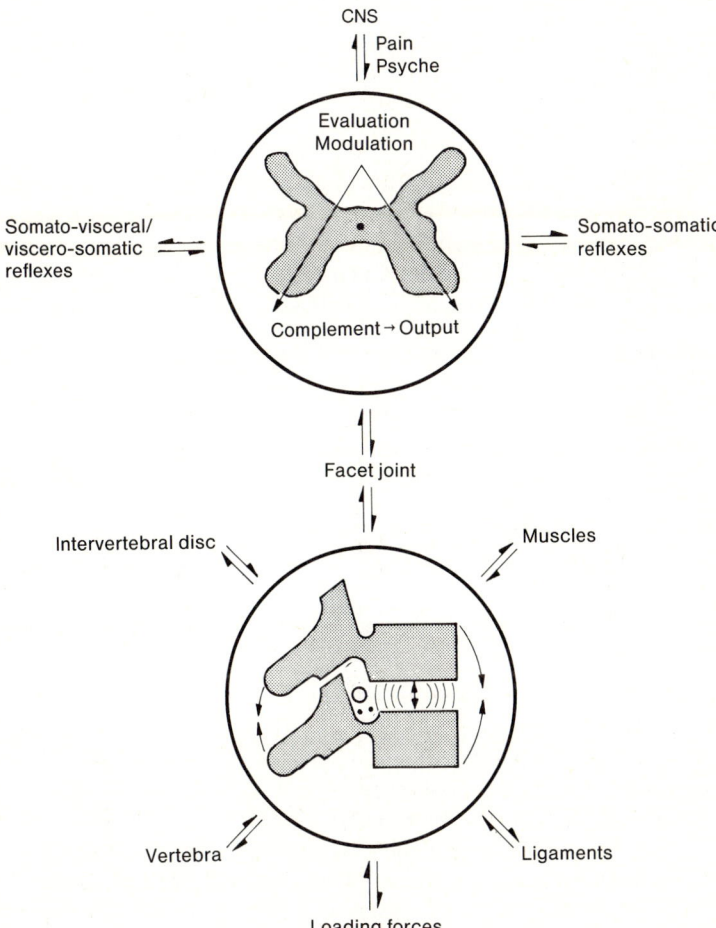

Fig. 1. The apophyseal joint shown in its dual function – *lower circle:* as part of the spinal segment and *upper circle:* as part of the reflexive neurologically mediated feedback mechanisms

2.2.1 Mechanical Circuit

Anatomically, the apophyseal joint is part of the spinal segment. The spinal segment is the smallest functional unit of the spine (Junghans 1954; please see Fig. 2). It consists of (1) the movable components: the intervertebral disc and the facet joint components; and (2) the stabilizing system: ligaments and muscles (Fig. 1 lower circle). Together, these two component systems form the actual functional unit. The core pressure of the intervertebral disc is the net (balanced) force between the various loading forces directed towards the spine (static loading, weight, etc.) and those forces exhibited by tissue tension (ligamentous elasticity and muscle tone of the spinal muscles, etc.).

This model will be used to illustrate the

- diagnostic and therapeutic approach
- clinical signs
- causes
- relative significance

of a somatic dysfunction (or functional disturbance) in the apophyseal joint.

A functional disturbance (somatic dysfunction) in a facet joint will lead to impairment in mobility in the other components of the spinal segment. In general, if one part of a spinal segment is involved, the remainder of that segment will also be affected as well. Thus, a somatic dysfunction in a facet joint, degenerative disc

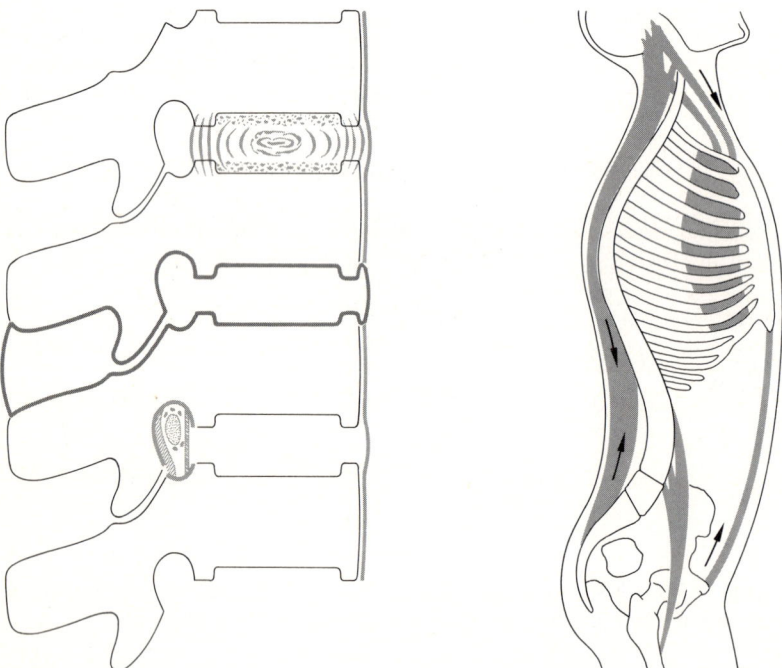

Fig. 2. The spinal segment – the smallest movable unit in the spinal column. (After Junghans 1954)

disease, ligamentous insufficiency and muscle imbalance associated with that joint all can either be the cause or the result of each other (Fig. 1, lower circle).

In addition to the segmental changes that can occur, the mechanical functioning of one spinal segment influences and is influenced by the overall loading and other mechanical forces of the spine and extremities (Fig. 3). For example, a leg length difference, extremity joint restriction, pelvic asymmetry, and trunk muscle tone changes all can lead to segmental changes and somatic dysfunctions. Conversely, segmental changes can affect the overall static and dynamic loading forces, as is seen with a compensatory and painful scoliosis due to an acute somatic dysfunction, for instance.

2.2.2 Nervous System and Reflex Circuit

The upper portion of Fig. 1 illustrates the various reflexes as they relate to the facet joint and the dermatome, myotome, CNS, vascular system, and internal organs. Similar to any other joint, the apophyseal joint has a large number of nerve endings in its joint capsule as well as in the associated ligaments and muscles. The

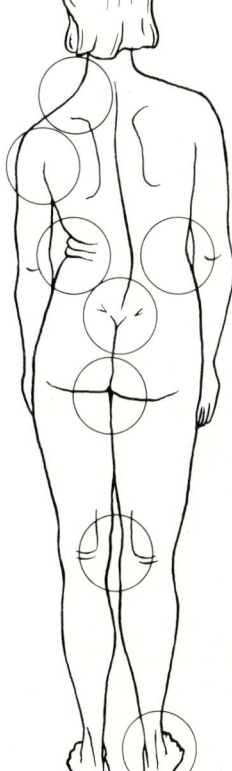

- asymmetry of the shoulders
- scoliosis
- asymmetry at the lumbo – sacral junction
- functional problems at the joints in the leg
- leg length differences

Fig. 3. Surface landmarks helpful in the static examination of posture

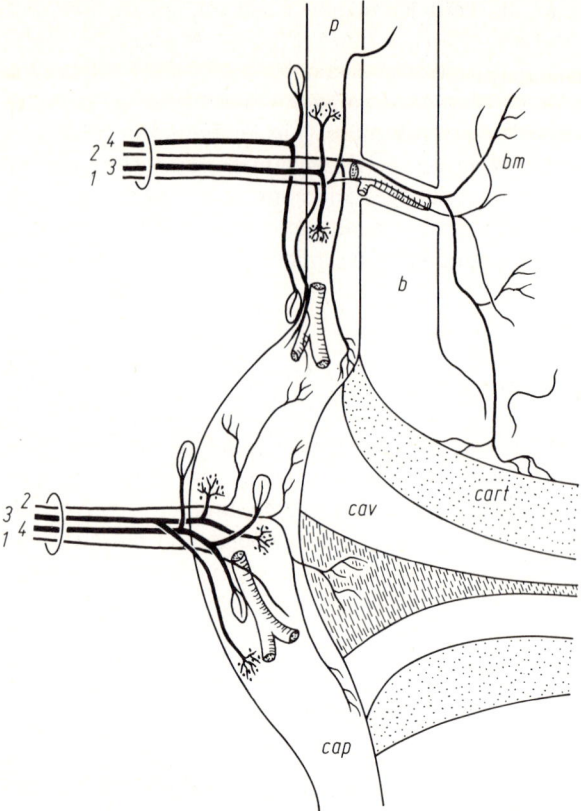

Fig. 4. Schematic representation of joint innervation. Afferent: *1* free, unmyelinated, thread-like nerve endings (type IV); *2* free fusiform nerve endings (type I); *3* receptors in clusters (type II); *4* encapsulated receptors (type III); *cap* joint capsule; *cav* joint cavity; *cart* cartilage; *b* bone; *bm* bone marrow; *p* periosteum. (After Polacek 1966)

nerve endings can be divided into two major groups: the proprioceptors, that is receptors I, II, III, and the nociceptors, the IV receptors. Due to the scope of this book, we would like to refer readers to the original papers by the various authors for a more detailed description of the anatomy and function of the receptors (Wyke and Polacek 1975, Fig. 4; Korr 1975; Wolff 1983; Dvořák and Dvořák 1983; Paterson and Burn 1986).

Proprioceptors convey information about body posture and joint position as they react to tension changes in the joint capsule, ligaments, tendons and muscles. The nociceptors are characterized by having a higher threshold than the proprioceptors and thus a stronger stimulus is needed, such as occurs with trauma, irritation or even inflammation of the joint capsule. Both proprioceptors and nociceptors relay the incoming message via the dorsal ramus of the spinal nerve to the posterior horn of the gray matter of the spinal cord. There, any change in tension or damage to the joint capsule is registered, interpreted, modulated (facilitation vs. inhibition) and stored. Once a certain threshold has been exceeded, the informa-

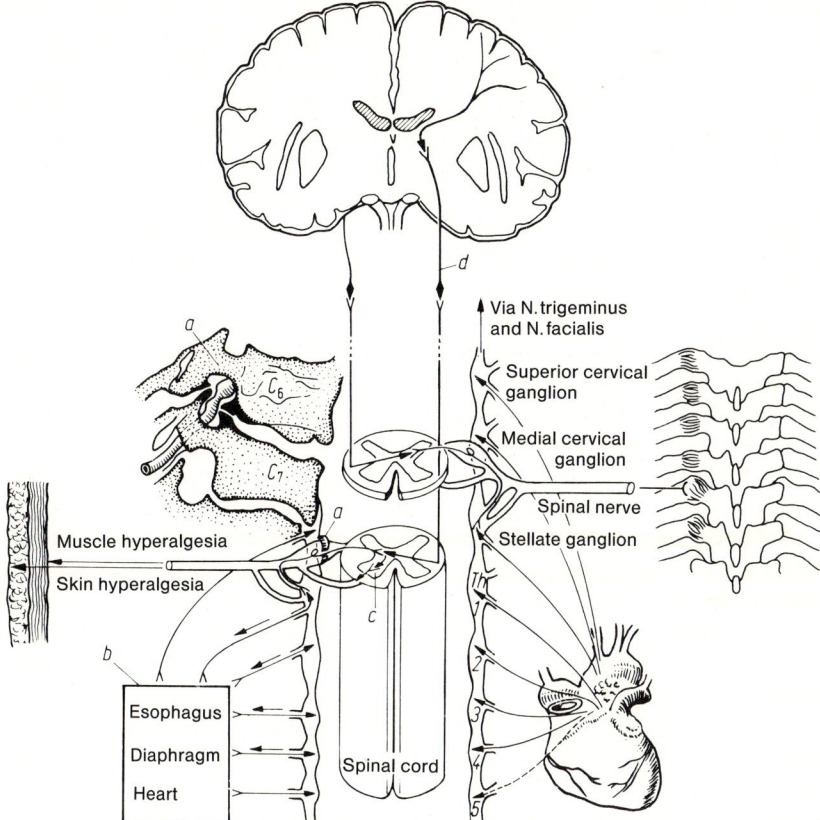

Fig. 5. The neuroreflexive relationships between the spine, CNS and internal organs. (After Kunert 1975)

tion, in one form or another, is relayed back to the periphery. Thus, a joint dysfunction has a marked influence on the short and long spinal muscles in the back and the muscles associated with the outer trunk and the extremities. Furthermore, it can have an influence on the skin and subcutaneous tissues, the vascular system and the viscera by altering reflexes associated with activity in the respiratory, cardiovascular and gastrointestinal systems. Once a certain threshold level has been exceeded, a somatic dysfunction may be reported to the CNS as pain or, especially if prolonged, may be accompanied by psychosomatic changes (Fig. 5).

Summation of different stimuli from various sources has been described by Korr (1975). A number of subthreshold stimuli may add up to reach a total suprathreshold level making apparent the otherwise unnoticed dysfunction. A so called "quiet" dysfunction often remains unnoticed until an additional stimulus is introduced either from a mechanical aberration or due to reflex changes associated with a faulty joint.

The goal of manual therapy is to both restore the mechanical function of a joint and normalize altered reflex patterns.

2.2.3 Practical Applications

The practical application is not as simple as the theory. The response to a somatic dysfunction in one spinal segment is primarily segmental in its distribution, but not entirely so. Some of the explanations include the following:

The joint capsule of a facet joint is innervated not only by the dorsal ramus of the spinal nerve that corresponds to the specific spinal segment but also by the rami from the spinal nerves above and below the segment in question (Wyke 1979). Also there are numerous modulation possibilities at the segmental level as well as at higher levels of the CNS. Variation is further enhanced by the influence of the efferent pathways via the radicular nerve fibers and the plexus systems, all of which can contribute to the variety of clinical symptoms. Thus, which muscle group or internal organ system is involved differs from case to case, even if the dysfunction is found to be at the same segmental level.

We have attempted to schematically present these rather complex processes in Fig. 1. The left half of the upper circle in the figure depicts the somato-visceral and viscero-somatic reflexes, whereas the right side shows the somato-somatic reflexes.

The **viscero-somatic** and the **somato-visceral reflexes** are mediated through the autonomic nervous system by way of the spinal nerves and communicating branches (Kunert 1975; Korr 1975) (Fig. 5). This reflex behavior may explain the interactions between somatic dysfunctions and subsequent changes at the internal organ level, and vice versa. This may explain the variety of **clinical presentations** possible (p. 88).

A thorough understanding of the **somato-somatic reflexes** is indispensable for **diagnosis** and **treatment**. Clinical practice has shown that it is useful to divide these reflex patterns into two major groups: those reflexes mediated through the *dorsal* ramus of the spinal nerve and those mediated through the *ventral* ramus.

The muscles innervated by the *dorsal* ramus are the so called autochthonous muscles of the back, that is the long and short muscles of the back. They are usually contracted when there is a somatic dysfunction, and often in a pattern that points in the direction of the dysfunction. Palpation of the tissues often elicits changes such as bogginess and swelling in areas the patient reports as tender or, as in some cases, as extremely painful (p. 36).

> Segmental tender points (zones of irritation) can be aggravated or relieved by appropriate provocative movement in the facet joint.

The dorsal ramus of the spinal nerve not only supplies the long and short muscles of the back but also the skin in the back about a hand's width on either side of the spine at the level of the individual spinal nerve. The affected area may then show orange peel-like thickening, and may be hyperalgesic and/or hyperemic. The skin rolling test (Fig. 6), dermatome needle testing or even thermography may be positive when examining this so called "test strip," thus pointing towards the presence of a somatic dysfunction. Electrophysiological evaluation as presented by Triano (1979) may be helpful.

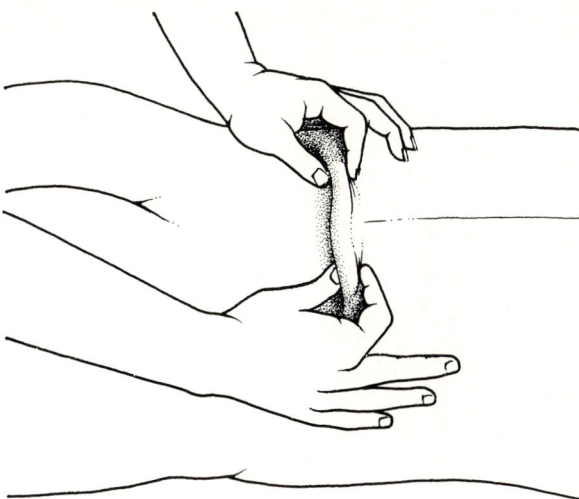

Fig. 6. Skin rolling test

> The tissue reaction mediated through the dorsal root is called *local* segmental irritation. It enables us to directly diagnose a somatic dysfunction.

The *ventral* ramus of the spinal nerve supplies the antero-lateral muscles of the trunk, the superficial layers of the back muscles and the muscles of the extremities and the associated skin zones.

The irritation may therefore appear quite distant from the point of origin of the dysfunction but should always be related to the corresponding segmental distribution. The localization of a segmental dysfunction in an extremity is facilitated by using the so called identification muscles (also known as indicator muscles; Hansen and Schliack 1962) (Fig. 7). These muscles, when involved, often demonstrate increased tone, a hardened palpable band ("myogelosis") or even tendomyositis and weakness.

Again these palpatory findings should aid in the diagnosis of a somatic dysfunction. The respective skin areas are often thickened and hyperalgetic (p. 52).

> The tissue reactions found in the peripheral muscles mediated through the ventral ramus of the spinal nerve are known as *peripheral* segmental irritation.

It should be emphasized that the pathways described here can be involved reciprocally. That is, any of the implicated structures, i.e. facet joint, ligaments, mus-

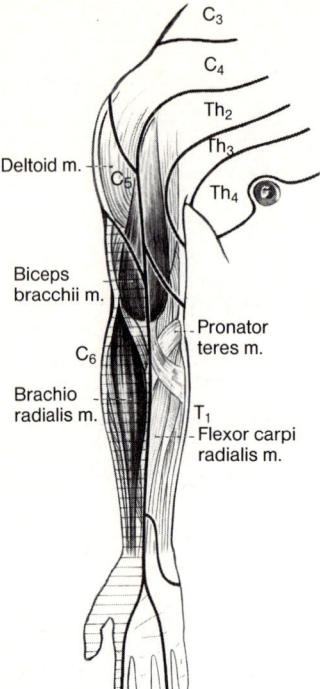

Fig. 7. Identification muscle. C6: paresis (but never complete atrophy!) of the biceps brachii and the brachioradialis muscles. (From Hansen and Schliack 1962)

cles, skin and soft tissue structures, vessels, viscera, or the CNS can either cause or be affected by a disturbance. Based on the understanding of these feedback mechanisms, manual medicine has freed itself from thinking in purely mechanical terms.

2.2.4 Diagnostic Signs of Somatic Dysfunction

In summary, a somatic dysfunction can lead to one of the following two disturbances:

1) joint motion restriction (see Fig. 1, lower circle), please also refer to p. 38,
2) disturbance in the neuroreflexive feedback mechanisms (see Fig. 1, upper circle).
   This may manifest itself as
   a) localized, segmental irritation (long or short muscles of the back, connective tissues, skin, etc.), p. 46,
   b) peripheral segmental irritation (peripheral muscles, segmentally related dermatomes), p. 52.

2.2.5 Causes of a Somatic Dysfunction

The information presented in Fig. 1 shows that there are four potential types of cause for a somatic dysfunction:

1) direct,
2) indirect, mechanical influences (lower circle),
3) indirect, neuroreflexive feedback mechanisms (upper circle),
4) combination of the above causes.

1): Direct causes. Somatic dysfunctions can result from one single faulty movement, such as incorrect turning when driving backwards in a car, missing a step while ascending or descending, or during sport activities. Further causes are inappropriate lifting of loads, as may occur when not bending the knees while lifting an object from the ground, with simultaneous turning of the spine; and faulty sleeping posture, especially when there is ligamentous insufficiency as is often seen in children.

2): Indirect, mechanical causes. Frequently a somatic dysfunction is due to faulty loading forces arising from vertebral asymmetries, intervertebral disc degeneration, pelvic asymmetries, leg length differences, motion restriction in the large joints, and foot deformities. Another important mechanical cause is muscle imbalance which may result from weakening or shortening of certain muscle groups and overall abnormal postural stress along with ligamentous insufficiency. Also, abnormal demands placed on the body structure due to non-physiological posture at work are a potential cause.

3): Indirect, neuroreflexive feedback mechanisms. Mediated through segmental reflex feedback mechanisms, a somatic dysfunction may result from a nociceptive reaction associated with a primary disturbance in a myotome, dermatome, the vascular system, an internal organ or psychological factors (Wolff 1983). The somatic dysfunction in this case can be due to a somato-somatic reflex (i.e. the original disturbance is in the muscle) or a viscero-somatic reflex, where the original localized visceral stimuli produce patterns of reflex response in segmentally related somatic structures (for example, a stiff shoulder as related to cardiac disease). Two more reflex patterns have been identified. In the somato-visceral reflex, localized somatic stimulation produces patterns of reflex response in the segmentally related visceral structures. In the viscero-visceral reflex, which is also known as the viscero-somato-visceral reflex, localized visceral stimuli produce patterns of reflex response in the segmentally related visceral structures.

4): Naturally any of the above causes can exist either singly or in any combination. The various nociceptive afferent stimuli can then summate and lead to a somatic dysfunction.

> In addition to identifying the possible cause or causes of a somatic dysfunction it is important to establish the *significance and role* the dysfunction at hand plays in the overall musculoskeletal functioning. It is the key to determining a successful therapeutic approach.

3 Diagnosis in Manual Medicine

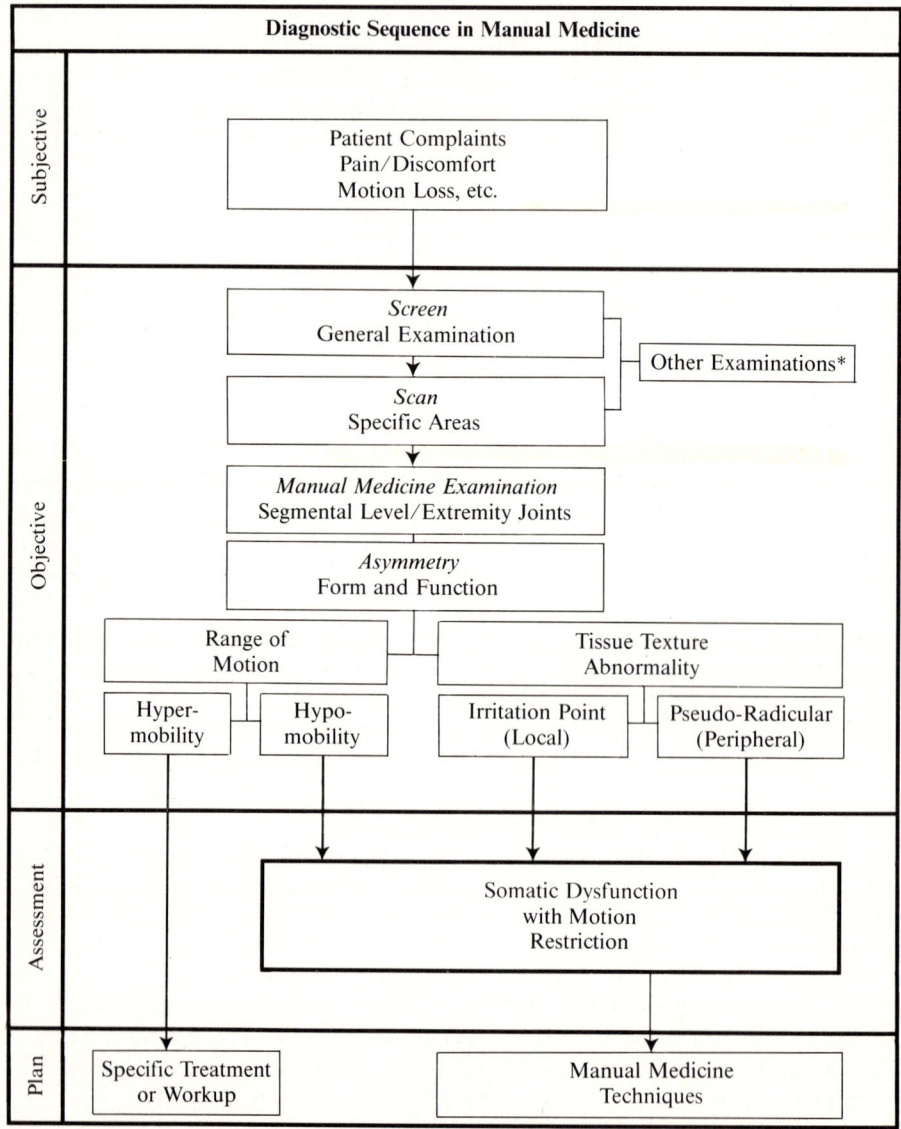

* As indicated for further workup.

3.1 General Evaluation

The diagnostic workup in manual medicine makes use of all those procedures that help detect reversible functional disturbances in the musculoskeletal system. The first step in assessing the patient is the routine history and physical examination, which provides a general impression of the patient's overall health status. With specific manual diagnostic techniques one will then be able to refine the routine static and dynamic examination of the musculoskeletal system. One can then, both quantitatively and qualitatively, detect even the most subtle motion deviations. Furthermore, with palpation certain reflexive changes can be detected that express themselves in tissue changes of the muscles, ligaments, subcutaneous tissues or skin.

Various approaches can be utilized to structure the diagnostic workup and formulation of a treatment plan. As in other fields of medicine, the problem oriented approach has been found very useful when dealing with a patient presenting with neuro-musculo-skeletal problems. The *SOAP* (Subjective, Objective, Assessment, Plan) format has proven quite practical, and to facilitate a better understanding of the approach used in the field of manual medicine, an overview is presented in the preceding algorithm (see p. 14).

Subjective data (i.e. symptoms) include the patient's chief complaint(s), history of the chief complaint, past medical or surgical history, allergies, medication use, and social and family history.

Objective data (i.e. signs) are those obtained through the physical examination as well as laboratory studies and adjunct tests. In manual medicine, after the appropriate history and general physical examination, the task of the initial examination is to search for findings of a somatic dysfunction in the various body regions. This more general examination has been referred to as *the screen* (Sect. 3.2). This is followed by *the scan* (Ward et al. 1981), which is an intermediate, more detailed examination of specific body regions and which focuses more on the segmental areas for further definition (Sect. 3.3). The *segmental manual medicine examination* is the final step in arriving at a specific segmental diagnosis (Sect. 3.4).

A way to remember which comes before which may be by the comparison to a screen door. One has to go through the screen door first before being able to enter the house. The acronym *ART*, representing the terms asymmetry, range of motion restriction, tissue texture abnormality, refers to the three specific changes associated with a somatic dysfunction.

If the criteria for a somatic dysfunction with motion restriction have been fulfilled (assessment) one can proceed to the next step, the therapeutic plan. If hypermobility was found the appropriate workup and/or treatment plan is to be initiated. Naturally, if at any time during the course of the history or examination other specific (i.e. neurologic or orthopedic) examinations are indicated, the appropriate workup must be followed.

A thorough understanding of the anatomy, biomechanics (White and Panjabi 1978), and neurophysiology (Wolff 1983; Wyke and Polacek 1975; Korr 1975; Dvořák and Dvořák 1983) is indispensable for a successful diagnosis.

3.2 General Manual Medicine Diagnosis (the Screen, Gross Manual Examination)

3.2.1 Surface Orientation

Exact landmark orientation on the body's surface is absolutely essential for a precise description of the diagnostic findings, evaluation of one's treatment success, and the ability to compare one's own work to that of other examiners. To this end, a series of landmarks or reference points have been identified for both the spinal column and the extremities.

3.2.1.1 Landmarks on the Extremities

The localization of landmarks on an extremity is actually rather simple.

The landmarks palpated in the shoulder girdle include: sternoclavicular joint, acromioclavicular joint, coracoid process, lesser and greater tubercle of the humerus, bicipital groove, superior and inferior angles of the scapula, and joint of the first rib (Fig. 8).

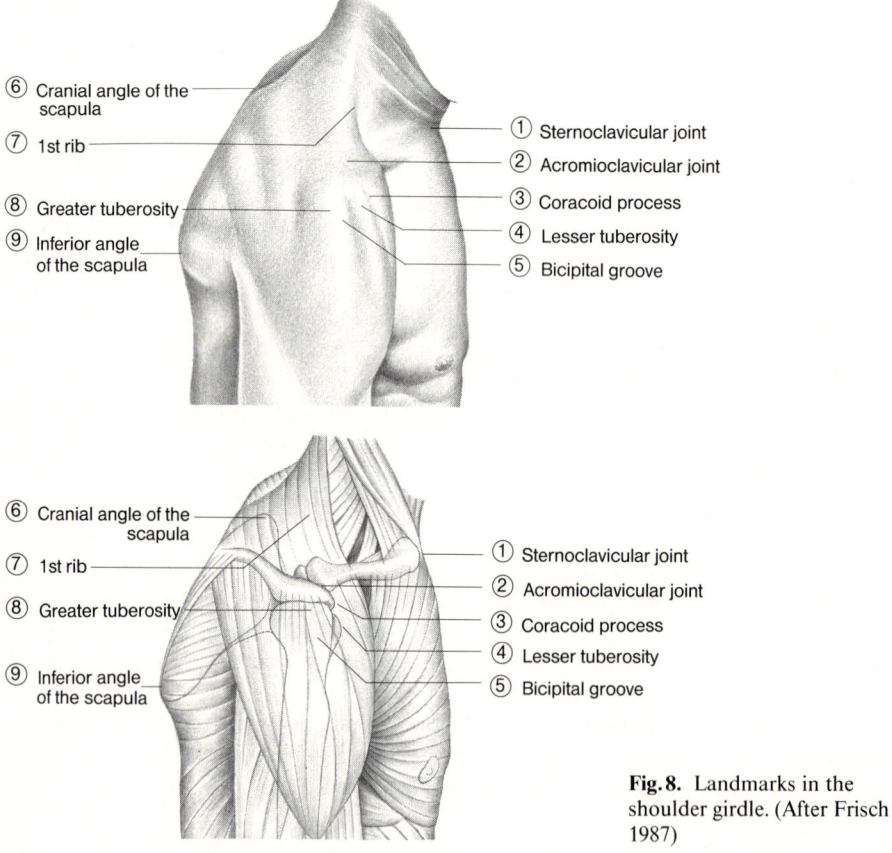

Fig. 8. Landmarks in the shoulder girdle. (After Frisch 1987)

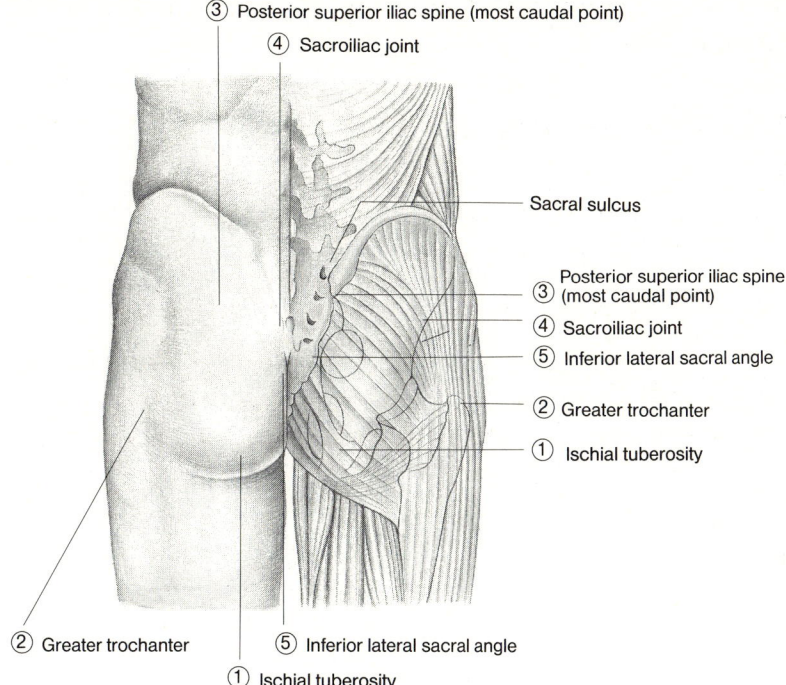

Fig. 9. Landmarks in the pelvic girdle. (After Frisch 1987)

Landmarks for the pelvis include the following (Fig. 9): ischial tuberosity, greater trochanter, posterior superior iliac spine, sacroiliac joint and inferior lateral sacral angle.

3.2.1.2 Landmarks on the Spine

It requires more skill to correctly and quickly identify the different landmarks on the cervical, thoracic and lumbar spine.

3.2.1.3 Landmarks on the Cervical Spine (Fig. 10)

C1: The transverse processes of the atlas can be palpated between the ascending ramus of the jaw and the mastoid process.
C2: Uppermost palpable spinous process of the cervical spine.
C5: First prominent spinous process to become palpable following the cervical lordosis from superior to inferior.
C7: In the unimpaired person, C6 moves anteriorly with respect to C7 with increasing cervical spine extension, allowing localization of C7.

In daily practice it is often not easy to exactly localize C7, as it is not always the most prominent vertebra.

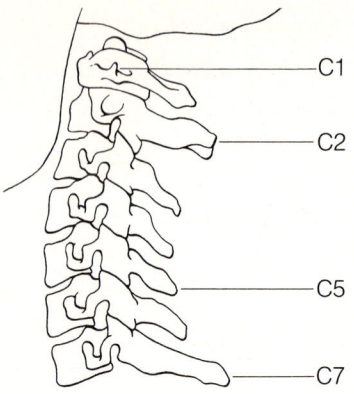

Fig. 10. Landmarks on the cervical spine (please refer to text)

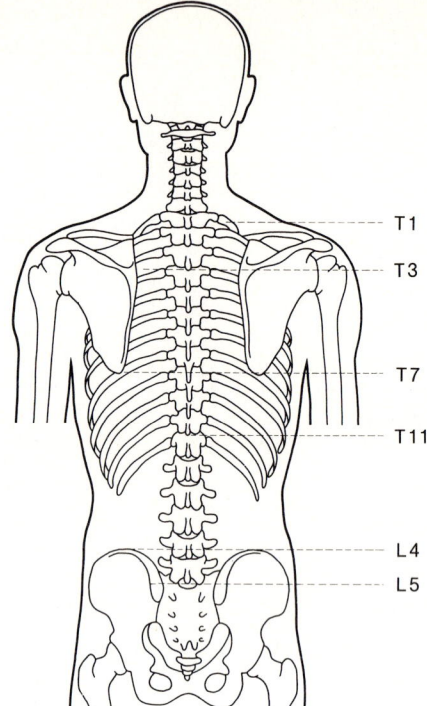

Fig. 11. General level orientation on the spine (please refer to text)

3.2.1.4 Landmarks on the Thoracic and Lumbar Spine (Fig. 11)

Gross orientation:

T1: The most inferior point of T1 can be localized by following an imaginary line straight through the sternoclavicular joint (Sell).
T3: Upper spine of the scapula with arm hanging at side.
T7: At the level of the inferior angle of the shoulder blade.
T11: Follow the most inferior rib pair medially.
L4: Approximately at iliac crest level.
L5: At the level of the center of the posterior superior iliac spine.

For more precise localization, Sell (Bischoff 1988) describes a series of additional landmarks, which, for didactic reasons, he calls "stations" (Fig. 12).

Sell first localizes C7. He then finds T5, T10 and T12 by counting the spinous processes, marking them at their most inferior portions. He selected these vertebrae in particular, because the distance between the most inferior portion of a spinous process and the corresponding facet joint is rather variable.

The most inferior point of the L5 spinous process can be localized by finding the midpoint of a horizontal line that has been constructed between the center of both posterior superior iliac spines (PSIS). To find the center of the PSIS, one first outlines its oval form with a pen and then divides it horizontally. The examiner can then start out from each "station" (C7, T5, T10, L12, L5) and localize the other spinal levels quickly.

General Manual Medicine Diagnosis

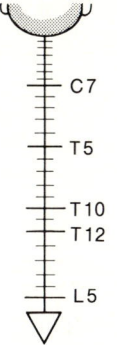

Fig. 12. Level orientation at the spine according to Sell (documentation scheme)

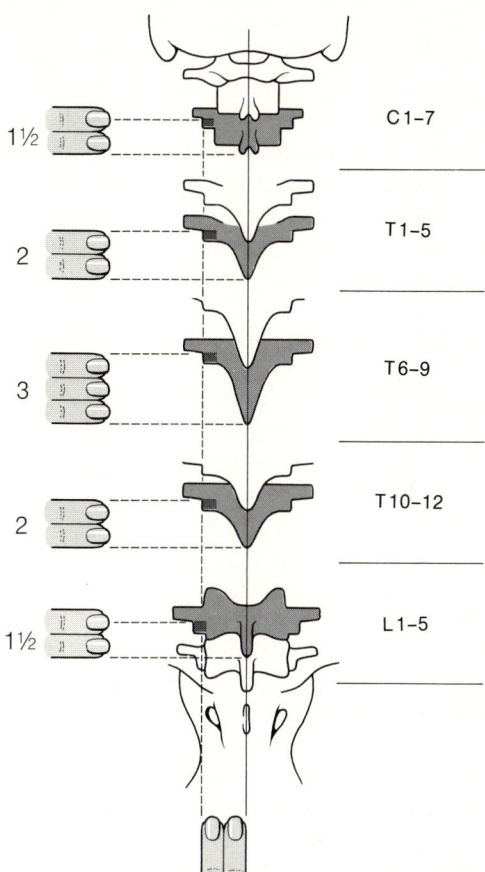

Fig. 13. The space between the facet joint and the most inferior point of the tip of the spinous process of the same vertebra in the various areas of the spine. (Drawing after Forte 1981)

Of utmost importance for manual diagnosis and therapy is the correct determination of the distance between the most inferior point of a spinous process of the vertebra in question and its related facet joint. This distance varies from spinal region to spinal region, and Sell recommends measurement utilizing finger widths (Fig. 13).

3.2.2 Layer Palpation

After the general identification of the surface landmarks, the examining hands palpate the deeper tissues. Again, palpation is a skill that requires constant practice and proper training so as to be able to utilize this sensory organ to the fullest (Beal 1967).

The student of manual medicine must learn the following:
- to palpate and evaluate the normal tissue structures such as the skin, fascia, muscles, ligaments and bone. Good handcare is absolutely necessary. Calloused fingers will have difficulty registering the more subtle changes;

- to feel and assess tissue changes by palpation;
- to recognize differences in quality, range and endfeel of joint movement;
- to evaluate postural asymmetry, both by inspection and palpation;
- to develop a three dimensional concept of anatomy and motion in space. While one of the physician's hands rests over the body area that is to be examined, the other hand moves the patient. The examiner receives a flow of information from both hands, trying to register the findings in as objective a manner as possible. The integrated information is then returned to the patient in form of the therapeutic intervention. Thus patient and physician form one "functional unit";
- to use palpation to detect the changes that occur with the treatment procedure.

During the examination both the patient and physician should assume a comfortable position. The examiner must concentrate hard during the examination so as to adequately register and assess the palpated information.

The following exercise was described to me by Greenman (personal communications 1983). It has proven to be very useful for developing palpatory skills in the assessment of tissue structures as well as joint movement.

Two persons sit opposite each other with their forearms resting comfortably on the table. The right hand of each person is designated the examining hand. The left arm of each person becomes the object to be examined. With the forearms resting prone on the table, each person places the entire right hand (palm and fingers) onto the forearm of the other person, just below the elbow.

1) The right hand makes slow and gentle contact with the skin. At first, the examining hand remains stationary, concentrating on the skin alone. The examiner thinks "skin," asking how thick, warm, cold, rough or soft is it? The left arm is then supinated. The examiner's right hand now evalutes this surface in a similar fashion and then compares the dorsal and volar surfaces with each other. Is there a difference in thickness, warmth, softness? Where? This limited, yet very concentrated, palpatory exercise involving the skin only makes it possible already to discriminate differences between the two arm surfaces.

2) Probing more deeply, so as to assess the subcutaneous tissues, the palpating hand (right hand) presses now somewhat more firmly onto the skin while moving the tissues back and forth both horizontally and longitudinally. We concentrate now only on the subcutaneous tissues. How loose or tight is it? In which direction can it and the overlying skin be displaced more easily. How thick is the layer? Tissue changes occurring as a result of a somatic dysfunction can often be found at this tissue level.

Now we take our watches off and feel the difference in consistency (more bumpy) and tissue thickness and compare this with the bare adjoining skin. Again, the tissue changes thus palpated are not unlike those often found in patients with somatic dysfunction.

3) In the subcutaneous tissues the course and direction of veins, nerves, arteries can be palpated.
4) Slowly, we increase the palpatory pressure until we feel the deep fascia encasing the deeper structures. Now we think "deep fascia," which may be de-

scribed in terms of firmness, softness and continuity. Moving our palpating hand gently horizontally across the forearm we palpate the deep fascial layer, and we notice the areas of thickening formed by the septa encasing the individual muscle bundles. The ability to recognize these muscle septa not only helps us differentiate between the individual muscle bundles but also aids in the localization of those structures lying deeply between the muscles.

5) While palpating the deep fascial planes we also start to concentrate on the muscles beneath. By focusing our attention we are then able to discern the muscle fibers and the direction in which they run.
We both now slowly open and close our left hands, allowing the forearm to relax and tense muscles. One should be able to recognize the difference with palpation. Next, we make as hard a fist as possible, again evaluating muscle changes during this activity. What we palpate at this point is similar to a "hypertonic" muscle, the texture of which is not unlike that palpated in muscles contracted secondary to a somatic dysfunction.

6) We continue the exercise by moving more distally, following the muscle layer until we notice a change in the tissue and can no longer feel muscle fibers. We are now at the muscle-tendon junction, the area where a muscle is most prone to injury.

7) Moving further distally beyond the muscle-tendon junction and towards the wrist, we can palpate a soft, rounded, smooth structure, the tendon. We evaluate the difference between muscle and tendon as well as the junction itself.

8) Staying at the same depth, the palpating hand continues to move again more distally. We encounter the transverse carpal ligament which holds together the tendons of the wrist. What are its characteristics? What is the course of its fibers? How thick is it? How firm? The ligaments in other portions of the body are similar when palpated.

9) We now return to the elbow with our palpating hand, placing the middle finger into a small groove on the dorsal side of the elbow. The thumb comes to rest on the opposite side on the volar side and palpates the radial head. We now concentrate on the bone, thinking "bone." Again we ask, how hard is it? What does the surface feel like? How does it react to pressure?

10) The index finger and thumb are now moved more proximally until they drop into the joint space. There is now a tissue structure beneath our fingers which under normal, healthy conditions should not be felt. This is the joint capsule which in most instances can only be palpated when there is a pathological change. Pathological alterations are in general not seen with a somatic dysfunction. Some of our colleagues maintain that once a joint capsule can be palpated, manipulative therapy is contraindicated (with the possible exception of the knee joint).

11) Thumb and index finger rest over the joint space. The left forearm is slowly and actively pronated and supinated, whereby one can feel the physiological barrier, which represents the end or limitation of the active range of motion. The same movement is repeated passively. In contrast to the active range of motion, this passive motion testing reveals information about the anatomical

barrier. Testing should be performed in succession, i.e. active followed by passive, but not alternating repeatedly passive and active movement.

Furthermore, this evaluation will aid in the assessment of joint resiliency, also known as "joint end-feel" (p. 28).

At this point, one should be reminded of the three most common errors encountered with inappropriate palpatory technique: lack of concentration, excessive pressure and too much movement.

To sum up, we have now palpated the skin, subcutaneous tissues, blood vessels, nerves, fascia, muscles, muscle-tendon junctions, tendons, ligaments, bones, joint space and the physiological and anatomical barriers.

The same structures that can be palpated on our forearms are found throughout our body. So, if in the clinical setting for instance, a patient complains about pain between the shoulderblade and the upper thoracic spine, layer palpation is useful in determining whether there is connective tissue swelling in the skin layer, muscle spasm in the trapezius muscle, tendinosis of the levator scapulae muscle, localized increased muscle tone of the long and short muscles of the back associated with vertebral or rib somatic dysfunction, or a process involving the bone itself.

The correct use of layer palpation is absolutely essential for accurate manual diagnosis of dysfunctions of the spine and extremities. Again, it cannot be emphasized enough that mastery of palpation requires adequate training and extensive clinical practice. Only by practicing is one able to refine the palpatory skills necessary to come up with an accurate palpatory assessment.

3.3 Specific Examination by Manual Medicine Techniques (the Scan)

3.3.1 Biomechanical Considerations

3.3.1.1 Joint Movement

A thorough understanding of joint mechanics is a prerequisite for exact diagnosis and specific treatment.

A vertebra can move about three axes and in three planes:
Each movement can be subdivided into
3 angular motions, namely
- flexion and extension,
- rotation to either side (right and left),
- sidebending to either side (right and left),
and
3 translatory motions (movement tangential to the joint surfaces, the evaluation of joint play), namely
- anterior and posterior,
- lateral (right and left),
- superior and inferior (Fig. 14).

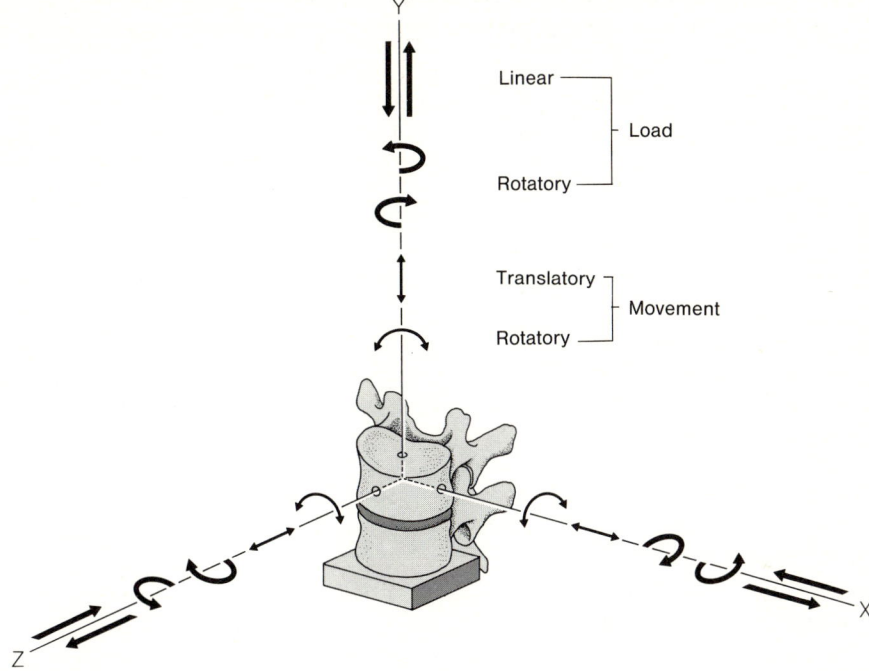

Fig. 14. The planes of vertebral motion utilizing a three-dimensional coordinate system. (After White and Panjabi 1978)

Conventionally, movement has been described as that of the superior vertebra in relation to the inferior vertebra. As reference point serves a point on the anterior superior surface of the vertebral body.

3.3.1.2 Range and Direction of Joint Movement

Range and direction of motion differ from joint to joint. The range of motion of a spinal joint is dependent on the intervertebral disc, the joint capsule and ligaments, provided the muscles are in a relaxed state. White and Panjabi (1978) have summarized such data (Table 1).

The *upper cervical spinal joints* represent an exception and area of special interest. The primary motion in the C0-C1 segment takes place about the transverse axis, that is 10° flexion and 25° extension. The sidebending and rotation movements can be detected by palpation as a springy movement. The primary motion in the C1-C2 segment is rotation, approximately 25° to either side (Fig. 15a, b).

The direction of movement in an apophyseal joint is the direct result of the joint surface inclination which varies from one spinal area to another. This is demonstrated in Fig. 16. In general, the joint surface arrangement changes gradually from a horizontal orientation (C0-C1, C1-C2, Fig. 15) through an oblique orientation (C2 through T11) to a vertical orientation in the lumbar spine (Fig. 16).

Table 1. Range of motion in the spinal segments C2 to S1

Spinal Segment	Flexion/Extension (rotation about X-axis) Range [degrees]	Mean	Sidebending (rotation about Z-axis) Range [degrees]	Mean	Axial Rotation (rotation about Y-axis) Range [degrees]	Mean
C2–C3	5–23	8	11–20	10	6–28	9
C3–C4	7–38	13	9–15	11	10–28	11
C4–C5	8–39	12	0–16	11	10–26	12
C5–C6	4–34	17	0–16	8	8–34	10
C6–C7	1–29	16	0–17	7	6–15	9
C7–T1	4–17	9	0–17	4	5–13	8
T1–T2	3–5	4	5	6	14	9
T2–T3	3–5	4	5–7	6	4–12	8
T3–T4	2–5	4	3–7	6	5–11	8
T4–T5	2–5	4	5–6	6	4–11	8
T5–T6	3–5	4	5–6	6	5–11	8
T6–T7	2–7	5	6	6	4–11	8
T7–T8	3–8	6	3–8	6	4–11	8
T8–T9	3–8	6	4–7	6	6–7	7
T9–T10	3–8	6	4–7	6	3–5	4
T10–T11	4–14	9	3–10	7	2–3	2
T11–T12	6–20	12	4–13	9	2–3	2
T12–L1	6–20	12	5–10	8	2–3	2
L1–L2	9–16	12	3–8	6	1–3	2
L2–L3	11–18	14	3–9	6	1–3	2
L3–L4	12–18	15	5–10	8	1–3	2
L5–S1	14–21	17	5–7	6	1–3	2

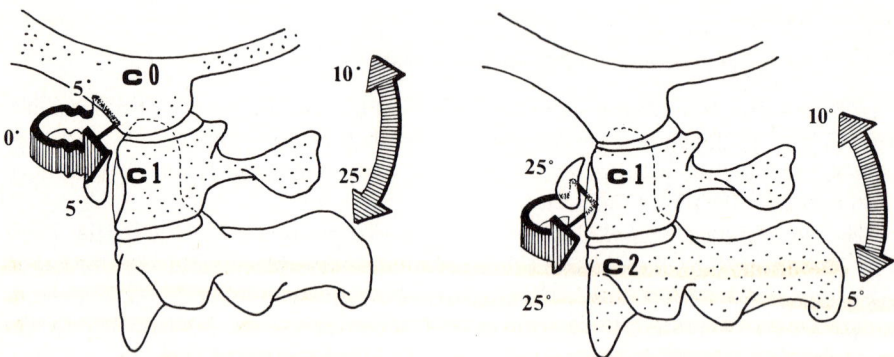

Fig. 15. Range of motion in the C0-C2 spinal segments. (After Kapandji 1970)

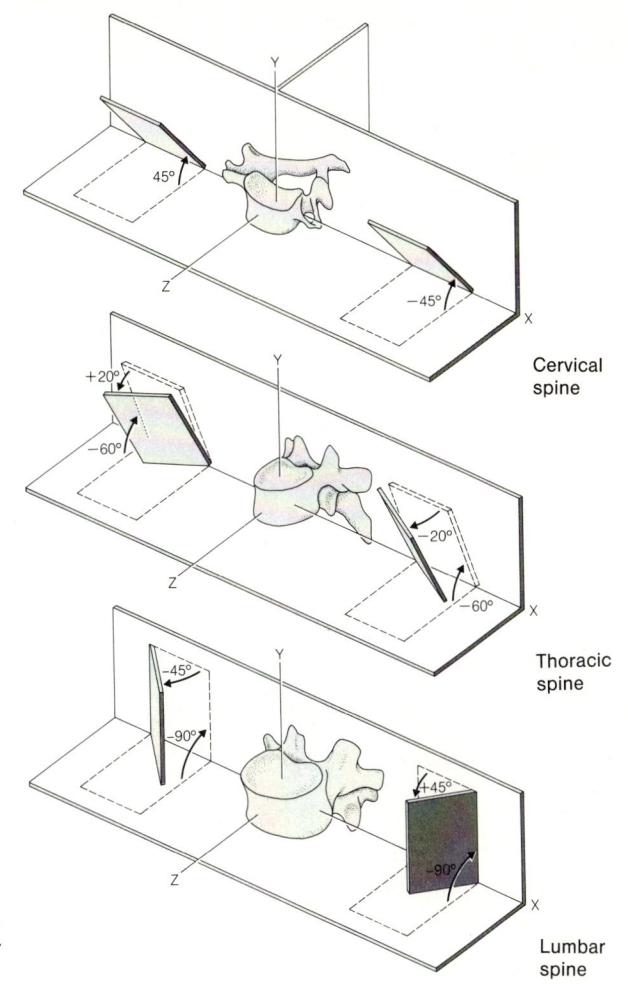

Specific Examination by Manual Medicine Techniques

Fig. 16. Graphical representation of the facet joint inclinations and axes of motion of representative vertebrae in the different spinal regions. (After White and Panjabi 1978)

Active isolated *sacro-iliac joint movement* is not possible. With lumbar flexion the sacro-iliac joint undergoes a small displacement, a motion that has been termed "nutation." At the S1 level the joint moves anteriorly whereas at the S3 level it moves posteriorly (Fig. 17).

Sacro-iliac joint movement becomes much more complex once the effects of the walking cycle come into play (Fig. 18). Take the case where the supporting leg (non-swing leg) is the left leg. The moment the left ilium glides posteriorly the sacrum starts to rotate about the right diagonal axis (which has been hypothetically constructed from the right outer angle of the sacral base to the left inferior sacral angle). The left sacral base thus moves anteriorly and inferiorly, while the right inferior angle of the sacrum moves posteriorly. On the right side, the swing side, the ilium rotates anteriorly as the leg swings posteriorly.

This sequence reverses when the swing leg moves anteriorly and the heel of the foot strikes the ground. Now the right leg becomes the supporting leg. The right

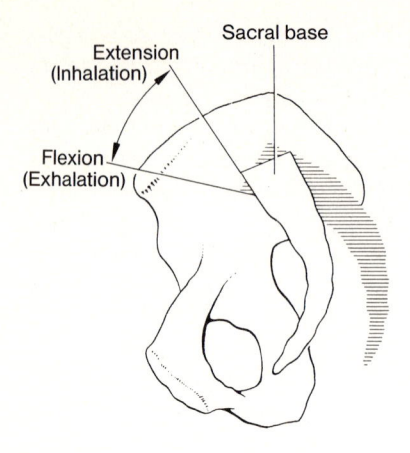

Fig. 17. The so called "nutation" movement of the sacrum

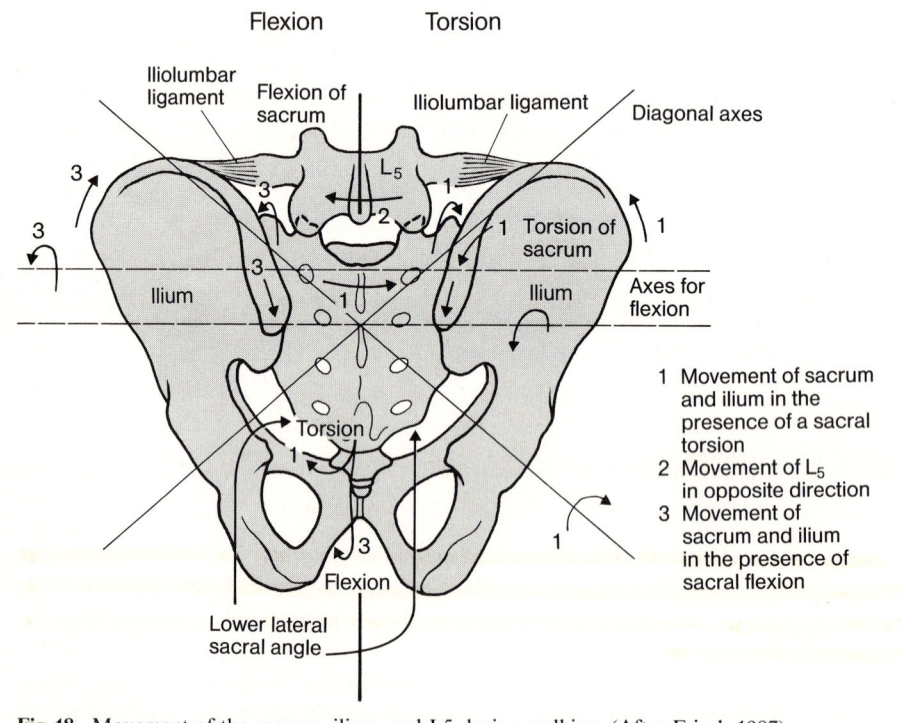

Fig. 18. Movement of the sacrum, ilium and L5 during walking. (After Frisch 1987)

1 Movement of sacrum and ilium in the presence of a sacral torsion
2 Movement of L_5 in opposite direction
3 Movement of sacrum and ilium in the presence of sacral flexion

ilium now swings posteriorly, and the sacrum rotates about the left diagonal axis. The left ilium rotatates anteriorly. Any of the described motion components can be impeded resulting in a dysfunction. Most common are dysfunctions related to the walking cycle, in contrast to the less frequent dysfunctions associated with pure forward bending. In addition, certain dysfunctions may be caused by trauma.

Specific Examination by Manual Medicine Techniques 27

In such cases, the joint movement does not follow along the normal, intrinsic physiological course, but instead may assume an entirely deviant path, as in the case where the whole semipelvis moves superiorly or inferiorly (see p. 99).

Naturally, the range and direction of motion in the *extremity joints* varies considerably. They may be classified according to the number of axes about which a joint may move. A joint may move about one, two or three axes.

An understanding of the function, form and structure of the individual joints is fundamental to diagnosis and treatment. A description of the individual extremity joints would be beyond the scope of this introductory book. For specific details, please be referred to the standard texts.

3.3.1.3 Range and Quality of Joint Motion

The Physiological, Anatomical, and Pathological Motion Barriers

Each joint can be moved actively within a certain limit or barrier. With the passive type of motion, i.e. that motion introduced by the examiner, one can carry the joint further to another limit or barrier, which also feels somewhat more firm at that point. The endpoint of the active range of motion is termed the physiological barrier, while the endpoint of the passive range of motion is known as the anatomical barrier. Motion between the physiological and anatomical barriers is the result of stretch and elasticity or resiliency in the soft tissues around the joint. This resiliency is palpated as a "springy" motion that becomes increasingly firm and tense when approaching the anatomical barrier. Kimberly (1979) has diagrammatically outlined these joint movements and barriers (see Fig. 19).

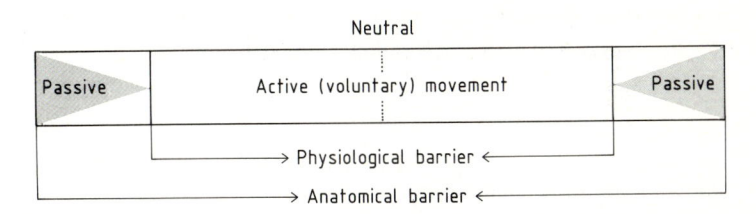

Fig. 19. Physiological and anatomical barriers

A joint with impaired function suffers a loss of mobility. In addition to the physiological and anatomical barriers in a normally functioning joint, there exists what has become known as the pathological barrier, which can restrict either active or passive movement or both.

Motion restriction may have several causes, one of which is a somatic dysfunction. The joint restriction can occur at any point along the normal range of motion.

A patient with a cervical spine dysfunction, where rotation to the right is restricted, for instance, holds his head turned to the left and may have difficulty turning the head back to the midline. This is often observed with acute dysfunctions and ones where onset was very recent. Kimberly has provided the diagrammatic representation shown in Fig. 20.

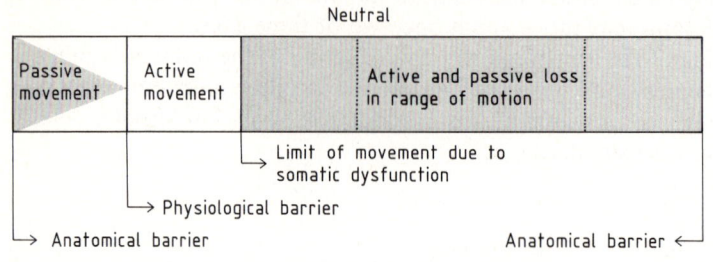

Fig. 20. Pathological barrier with acute somatic dysfunction

Minor motion loss, as encountered in rather chronic dysfunctions for instance, and where less than half of the range of motion is lost, can be represented as in Fig. 21.

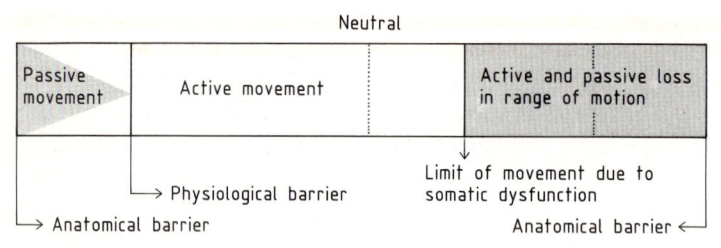

Fig. 21. Pathological barrier with chronic somatic dysfunction

It should be emphasized that these diagrams, for simplicity reasons, illustrate movement in one plane only.

Figure 22 demonstrates the application of these principles as related to the three planes of movement in a spinal segment.

Kimberly's diagrams are an excellent didactic tool in helping understand some of the principles important to the manual medicine examination and assessment of joint mobility.

End-feel

An additional and significant component in manual diagnosis is the palpatory assessment of the "end-feel," a concept introduced by Cyriax in 1969.

During the general examination of a joint, various qualities can be ascribed to the sensation perceived by the examiner at the motion barrier of a joint. With el-

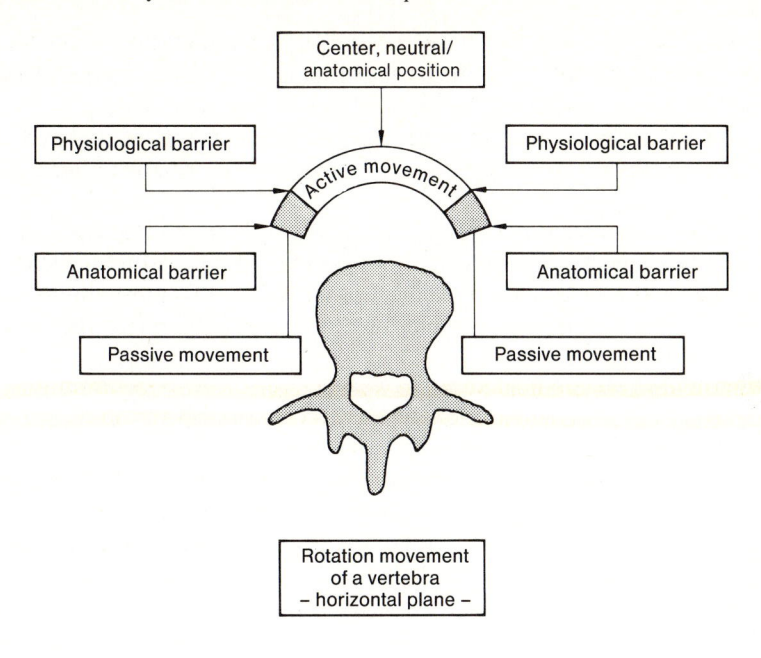

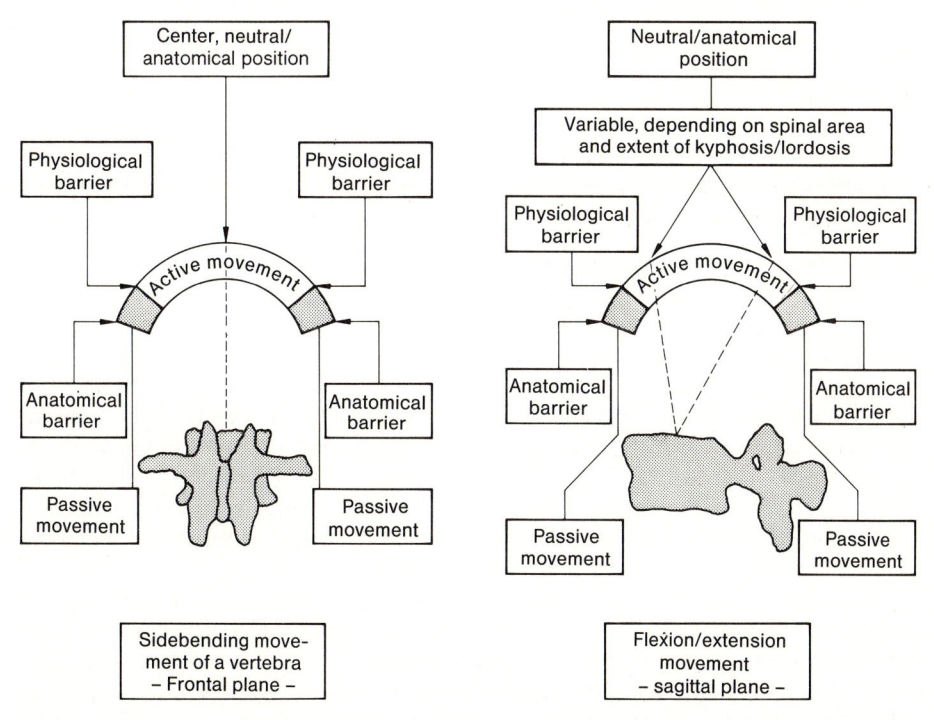

Specific Examination by Manual Medicine Techniques

Fig. 22. Model proposed by Kimberly for the angular vertebral motion along three axes of motion (rotation, sidebending, extension/flexion)

bow flexion, for instance, one palpates a rather soft and elastic end-feel which is due to muscle limitation. In contrast, with pronation and supination of the forearm one will palpate a firm-elastic end-feel due to ligamentous stop.

This again is to be contrasted to the hard-elastic end-feel encountered with elbow extension, where the barrier is due to bone to bone or bone to ligament interaction.

The manual examination evaluates the quality of both the angular and translational joint movements at the barrier. In a normal, unaffected joint the barrier in both angular and translational movement is sensed as soft. Furthermore, one can passively advance the movement from the physiological barrier to the joint's anatomical barrier (Fig. 19).

If a hard end-feel is palpated within the physiological range of motion, and if the joint cannot be carried further passively, a pathological end-feel is present (Figs. 20 and 21).

The end-feel associated with a pathological barrier assumes different qualities, thus being an important diagnostic indicator for different disturbances. The end-feel has been described as hard if there are bony changes, e.g. after trauma, as hard-elastic secondary to scar formation, or as firm-elastic because of muscle spasm or somatic dysfunction. Successful manual therapy normalizes the end-feel.

Kaltenborn (1976) points out that one may also encounter an "empty feel," that is no end-feel. This happens when the patient does not allow movement to the actual barrier because of pain associated with trauma, inflammation, or joint destruction or for psychological reasons.

Joint Play

Although there is no joint surface that is perfectly level or perfectly spherical, we will illustrate the mechanics of joint movement by utilizing the ideal case of two solid bodies moving against each other.

Movement can be broken down into the following categories:
a) gliding movement,
b) rotational (rolling) movement,
c) combination of rotation and gliding, the roll-gliding movement.

In gliding, one point on one surface shifts position relative to a stationary point on the other surface, covering a certain distance away from the starting point. Thus, the stationary point comes successively into contact with new points on the moving surface. This movement is associated with a lesser or greater loss of energy due to friction. However, friction is usually lessened by various lubrication methods, e.g. hydromechanical or electromechanical methods.

During rotational movement, the points of contact on both the level surface and on the curved surface change. The points which make contact with each other at one instant are replaced by two new points which come into apposition as the cylinder turns. Again, there is a certain distance covered, but in contrast to the gliding movement, there is relatively little energy lost with rotation. In technical applications, this is the preferred system, such as in ball-bearings, etc.

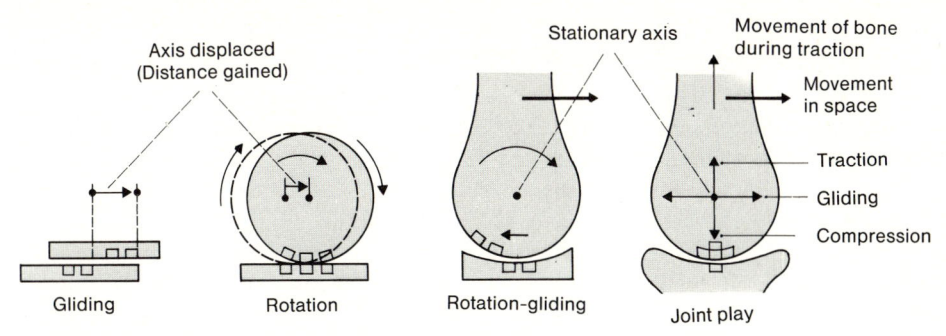

Specific Examination by Manual Medicine Techniques

Fig. 23. Movements possible between two solid bodies. (After Frisch 1987)

In the rotation-gliding movement, the axis of the rotating body remains fixed or stationary. In this case, as the axis of the moving body remains constant, the body does not cover any distance, similar to the gears in a clock, where the wheels turn but the axes remain fixed.

Most of the motion processes in biological systems are a combination of rotation and gliding movements. The anatomical arrangement of the joint surfaces determines the relative proportion of the rotational and gliding movements (Fig. 23).

For two solid bodies to be able to move in space there must exist some "room," space or "play" between them. The axle of a railway car or a cupboard drawer, for instance, can only move if they are not planted firmly against their support. There must be a minimum of mobility in directions other than the major functional directions inherent in the object's surface. For a drawer to be functional for instance, it must have sufficient room to move, albeit ever so small, in up-down and side-side directions, which is not related to the drawer's functional movement of forward and backward.

Similarly, each joint has some play in directions other than that of its functional movement. The "play" is made up of small gliding processes not contributing directly to the main direction of a joint's movement. In a normal, non-impeded joint, the examiner can feel a fine shifting of joint surfaces against each other, tangential to the plane of the joint, by moving one joint partner against the other stationary partner. Through the introduction of tractional forces, the examiner is able to lift one joint partner away from the other, by however little. The sum of all these passively introduced movements has been termed by Menell "joint play" (1952). Joint play is best assessed with the joint in its neutral position.

The following example should help in the understanding of what is meant by joint play.

Take a simple joint, the metacarpophalangeal joint, for instance. It can actively be flexed and extended to its extreme, the physiological barrier. Further passive extension and flexion should be possible, so as to bring the joint to its anatomical barrier. In addition to the functional direction of flexion and extension, one can move the joint partners in planes parallel and perpendicular to the tangential plane of the joint's surface.

In practice, the examiner brings the joint into its neutral position, where he/she then fixates the proximal joint partner, e.g. the head of the metacarpal bone. The

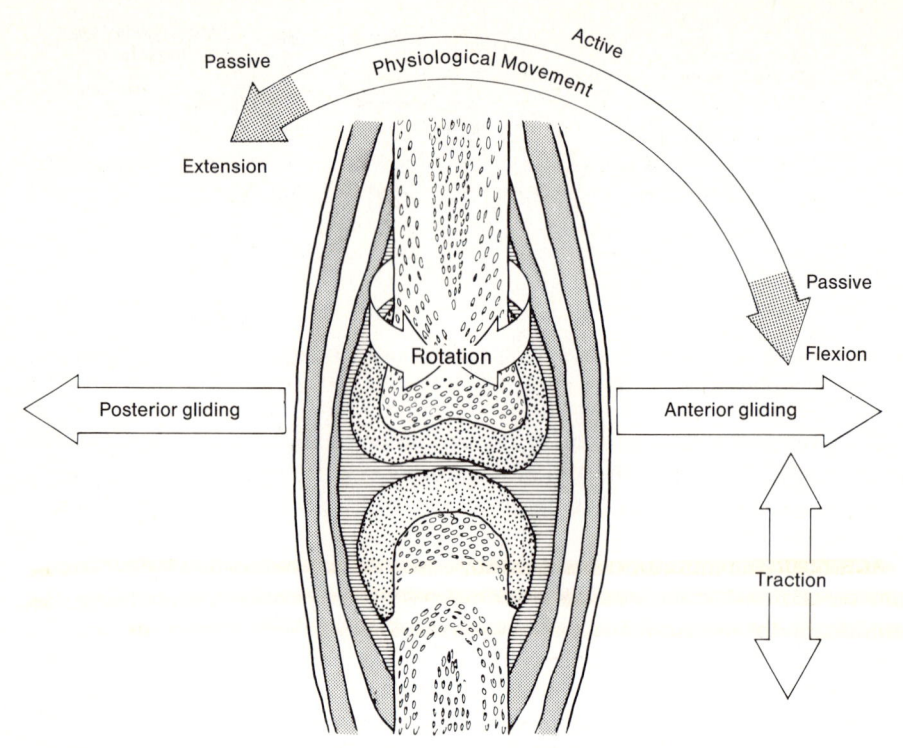

Fig. 24. Joint play as demonstrated at the proximal interphalangeal joint

distal partner, the phalangeal base, is then moved in planes parallel and perpendicular to the tangential plane of the joint. One can observe the following movements, as diagrammed in Fig. 24:

- parallel gliding movement of the joint surfaces against each other in the posterior-anterior direction,
- parallel gliding movement in the radio-ulnar direction,
- rotation about the longitudinal axis of the metacarpophalangeal joint,
- traction.

For a joint to function normally, sufficient joint play must be assured. In cases of dysfunction joint play will be diminished or in some cases even absent. One of the essential tasks of the diagnostic endeavor in manual medicine is to recognize the presence of joint play abnormalities. After establishing the specific manual diagnosis appropriate manual therapeutic intervention can be initiated.

3.3.1.4 Physiological Motion of the Spine: Fryette's Rules

Up to this point, we have only examined mobility in one single joint. We have to extend our discussion and take a closer look at how the joints function as a group in the different areas of the spine.

Flexion and extension are the only independent motion directions in the spine. Pure sidebending and rotation occur in a very limited fashion in a spinal segment as they are almost always coupled to each other. This means that there is no significant sidebending without simultaneous rotation, and vice versa.

Sidebending and rotation may be in the same direction or run in the opposite directions. The direction of the coupling of motion is a function of both the joint surfaces of the facet joints and the degree of flexion or extension of the spine.

Fryette has proposed the following three major principles describing the physiological motions of the spine (1954):

Rule 1: When the spine is in a neutral position, that is neither flexed nor extended, and sidebending is introduced, the bodies of the vertebrae will rotate towards the convexity. In other words, if the spine is in the neutral position, the direction of sidebending is always opposite that of rotation. Thus when sidebending is introduced to either a lumbar or thoracic vertebra, the same vertebra rotates towards the convexity, with the maximal rotation component being at the antero-posterior apex.

With the spine in the neutral position, the joint surfaces experience the least amount of loading force stress and the joint capsules the least amount of tension. The neutral position is only a small portion within the range of movement in the sagittal plane.

According to Fryette, the cervical spine is unable to assume a neutral position, as the joint surfaces are always subject to loading force stress along with continued tension at the joint capsules.

Rule 2: When the spine is either flexed or extended and sidebending is introduced, the vertebrae will rotate towards the concavity, that is to the same side.

Summarizing the first and second rules, one can make the following conclusions:
In the cervical spine, from C2 to C7, sidebending and rotation always occur in the same direction, independent of the degree of flexion or extension. The C0-C1 joint, however, is an exception due to its anatomical arrangement. There, sidebending and rotation take place in opposite directions.

In the thoracic and lumbar spine, sidebending and rotation are in opposite directions as long as the spine is in the small neutral range. That is sidebending to the right is associated with rotation to the left. When the spine is either extended or flexed, sidebending and rotation occur in the same direction. Thus, sidebending to the right will cause rotation to occur to the right as well.

Rule 3: Any movement of the spine will influence and modify all other movement components.

These principles are of great importance in daily practice. Rules 1 and 2 find their application in the preparation of the patient for specific, well localized manipulative intervention, as the slack must be taken out in the spinal segments next to the incriminated segment. The first rule in most cases plays less of a role, as the patient is almost always treated with the spine either in flexion or extension.

Slack is taken out by guiding the spinal segments next to the one in question into a direction exactly opposite to the physiologically coupled motion direction. For example, when the cervical spine is bent to the right side and rotated to the left, the facets on the right side of the apophyseal joints are compressed while on the left side the joint capsule and tendons are stretched. Thus, on the concave side, the facet joints are in the *"close packed"* position, with the ligaments on the left being stretched taut. Similarly, the slack is taken out in the remainder of the spine by moving the spinal areas next to the incriminated segment in a direction opposite that of the physiological coupled motion.

By careful extension and flexion of the spine one is able to precisely localize the incriminated segment and take out the slack in the adjoining segments.

Careful preparation and taking out the slack is demonstrated in the following example:

L2-L3 is found to be restricted. For simplicity reasons, the direction in which the restriction occurs will not be considered at the moment. The patient is brought into a right side-lying position and slight flexion is introduced to the spine. A pillow is placed under the lumbar spine which allows the thorax to undergo sidebending to the right. The operator's left hand is placed over the spinous process of L2, while the right hand is placed on the spinous process of L3. Now, the patient is rotated to the left through his thorax until movement is perceived at the level of the L2 spinous process. At the same time, the pelvis is rotated to the right until movement is perceived at the L3 spinous process. By this maneuver, the slack has been taken out above L2 and below L3. The incriminated joint, however, is not "locked" and is now ready to be treated

The third rule implies that the spine should best be examined in the neutral position, as the diagnostic findings are more precise in this position. Exact motion testing is more difficult when the patient is sitting either exaggeratedly erect (spine extended) or slouched forward (spine flexed), as part of joint mobility will be lost in favor of either flexion or extension.

3.4 The Segmental Manual Medicine Examination

First a word about terminology. One can describe a diagnostic finding in two ways, namely by reporting either the *position* of the components of a joint in relation to each other (static) or the joint *movement behavior* (dynamic). Thus, one can report that "the vertebra is flexed, sidebent to the right and rotated to the right." The same findings can be expressed in rather functional terms such as "the vertebra resists extension, rotation to the left and side-bending to the left."

In both cases we are dealing with the same findings. Confusion and misunderstandings come about when the various authors and practitioners do not clearly indicate which terminology they are using. However, as with many other subjects in which the terminology is subject to variation and new influences, once learned, it is easy to adjust and interchange.

The Segmental Manual Medicine Examination

> A somatic joint dysfunction can be diagnostically evaluated by one of the following three manual medicine techniques:
>
> 1. palpatory assessment of joint mobility,
> 2. palpatory assessment of localized segmental irritation,
> 3. palpatory assessment of peripheral segmental irritation.

Some investigators exclusively utilize joint mobility (Stoddard, 1970). Others rely primarily on local tissue reactions (Maigne 1961; Sell 1969) and/or peripheral tissue reactions (Maigne 1961; Sutter 1975; Brügger 1977). It has proven beneficial to be familiar with more than one examination technique. This is especially helpful when confronted by a difficult case, as the findings elicited through the various techniques can be compared with each other, contributing therefore to the diagnostic workup.

The *direction* and *extent* of motion restriction associated with a somatic dysfunction are diagnosed by testing *joint motion* (Sect. 3.4.1) and assessing the *local* segmental irritation (Sect. 3.4.2).

The *peripheral* segmental irritation (Sect. 3.4.3) is clinically useful as it is an indication of a disturbance in the segmentally related joint.

The Segmental Examination of the Spine Using Manual Medicine Techniques

Bischoff (1988) suggests a "3-step diagnosis," which, supplemented by recommendations from Stoddard (1961), is presented here.

The functional manual medicine diagnosis of the spine follows three steps:

1. Segmental motion testing	1. Indicates if there is hypomobility
2. Localization of irritation points	2. Indicates if there is "segmental irritation"
3. a) Motion testing after Stoddard b) Functional segmental irritation point diagnosis	3. Determines if manual therapy is indicated

The examiner should be familiar with the precise localization of the various vertebrae (p. 17). He/she must know exactly which spinal segment is involved.

The *first* step helps determine whether there is hypomobility (restriction in movement) or hypermobility (p. 85). If hypomobility is palpated at the incriminated segment it does not automatically mean that one is dealing with a somatic dysfunction. Hypomobility may also be caused by a ruptured disc, degenerative changes, inflammatory or other destructive processes as well as trauma. These latter causes must be excluded through a thorough clinical workup, which should always include a thorough physical examination and appropriate orthopedic and neurological evaluation as well as the necessary radiological and laboratory studies.

The *second* step evaluates whether the hypomobility at the involved spinal segment is accompanied by segmental irritation (p. 10). If there is segmental irritation, it is extremely important to always palpate the corresponding irritation point. The localization of the irritation point is described in detail in Sect. 3.4.2. The examiner must localize the nodular pea-sized, tissue reaction, which is associated with tenderness when palpated. It is the result of increased muscle tension in the deep musculature of the back and the associated swelling of the connective tissues around the joint.

The palpatory finding of a segmental irritation point in and of itself is not proof of a somatic dysfunction with motion restriction. Similar palpatory findings can be the result of decompensated hypomobility, spondyloarthritic irritation, etc.

The presence of hypomobility and segmental irritation may indicate that there is some disturbance affecting a joint but is not pathognomonic for a somatic dysfunction.

The *third* step, therefore becomes necessary for further differential workup. *Motion restriction* (joint hypomobility) due to a somatic dysfunction has the following characteristics: motion in the incriminated joint is never totally lost, but is more restricted in one direction than another. Joint play is always diminished, and the endfeel at the pathological barrier has undergone specific changes. With a good three dimensional understanding and a careful segmental examination along the three planes, the direction and extent of motion restriction can be exactly determined (flexion-extension, sidebending and rotation).

If the examination reveals motion restriction to be present in *all* three planes, the motion loss is *not* due to a somatic dysfunction. Causes other than a somatic dysfunction must be determined and one must refrain from using manual therapy in this situation.

The *segmental irritation point associated with* a somatic dysfunction differs from other irritation points in that the former is not "constant", that is, it changes as the joint is moved passively. Both tissue texture and tenderness are directly related to the position and direction in which the joint is being carried. When the restricted joint is passively guided towards the pathologic barrier (p. 28), the irritation point is more easily palpated (keeping the palpatory pressure constant) and is perceived by the patient as more painful. When carrying the joint away from the pathologic barrier the irritation point is less prominent on palpation and less tender. With these concepts in mind, each joint can be adequately evaluated along its three planes of motion so as to determine the exact direction and position in which the joint is restricted. A specific and adequate treatment plan can then be formulated.

When learning manual medicine examination techniques, the novice may find it confusing which of the many motion components, i.e. which of the motion directions, should be evaluated first. Greenman (1984) therefore recommends to start the examination by evaluating the flexion and extension components first.

In the healthy state, the superior components of the apophyseal joint move anteriorly with flexion of the spine, that is the joint "opens up." With extension movement of the spine, the superior facet joint partners move posteriorly, that is the joint "closes." Either one of these motion components can be restricted. Depending on whether the joint is restricted in extension or flexion, sidebending and rotation movements at that joint are affected as well, but in different directions. (It

The Segmental Manual Medicine Examination

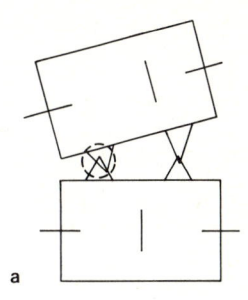

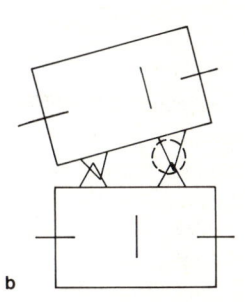

Fig. 25 a, b. Vertebral rotation to the right can be decreased by: **a** flexion restriction of the left facet joint – the irritation point can be palpated on the the left; **b** extension restriction of the right facet joint – the irritation point can be palpated on the right

may be useful to visualize these movement changes by using a skeleton as demonstration.)

If, say, flexion is restricted at the *left* facet joint, sidebending to the right and rotation to the right are also affected (decreased). If extension is restricted at the *right* facet joint, i.e. the joint partners do not approximate or do not "close," sidebending and rotation to the right are *also* restricted (Fig. 25 a, b).

Conversely, if there is flexion restriction at the *right* facet joint, sidebending and rotation to the left are restricted; with extension restriction of the *left* facet joint, sidebending and rotation to the left are *also* restricted.

These biomechanical relationships (flexion vs. extension restriction) may explain the fact that with vertebral rotation restriction to the right, for instance, the point of irritation can be found either on the right or left side. The former case is associated with an extension restriction of the right facet joint, and the latter case with flexion restriction of the left facet joint (Bischoff 1988) (Fig. 25 a, b).

Documentation/Record Keeping

Findings elicited through motion testing and localization of the irritation point can be represented either graphically or in abbreviated form.

Motion restriction at the C5–C6 segment can be indicated by drawing an arrow representing either flexion or extension, as well as sidebending or rotation. Transverse bars then are used to indicate the severity of the motion restriction, i.e. as follows:

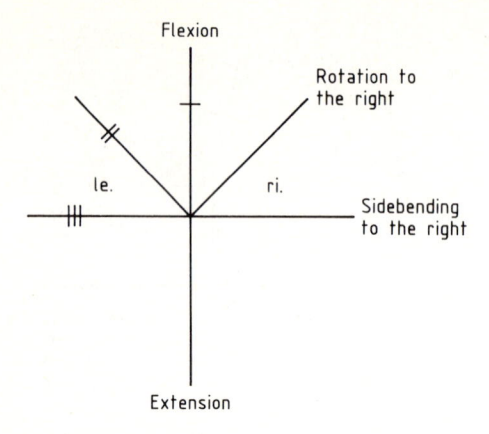

```
                Flexion
                   |
                   |    Rotation to
                   |  / the right
                \  | /
                 \ | /
             le.   |   ri.
                   |         Sidebending
        —|||——————————————  to the right
                   |
                   |
                   |
                   |            |   = somewhat limited
                   |            ||  = moderately limited
               Extension        ||| = significantly limited
```

Certain abbreviations have been utilized to describe similar findings. Thus the notation *C5–C6, right, FSB(Lt)R(Lt)* indicates that the facet joint between C5 and C6 on the right is restricted in flexion *(F)*, sidebending *(SB)* to the left *(Lt)* and rotation *(R)* to the left.

The irritation point can be indicated by a ± sign showing on which side it is palpated (in the above example on the right).

The following paragraphs will describe the motion testing examination procedure suggested by Stoddard and the localization of the various irritation points at the different spinal levels.

3.4.1 Palpatory Assessment of Joint Mobility (Motion Testing)

The palpating finger rests over the articular pillar and spinous or transverse processes of the spinal segment in question. One evaluates both quality and range of motion in that spinal segment in addition to any soft tissue changes. With the other hand, the examiner guides the patient's movements, thus assisting in the localization of the somatic dysfunction.

3.4.1.1 Cervical Spine – Motion Testing

C0–C1:

With passive sidebending, the ipsilateral transverse process of the atlas projects between the mastoid process and the superior ramus of the mandible (Fig. 27). It is important not to sidebend the entire cervical spine but rather introduce a nodding-like movement between the atlas and the occiput.

Rotation is rather minimal in the C0–C1 joint (Figs. 15 and 28). The cervical spine is passively rotated to its extreme, that is, one introduces rotation to the cervical spine until movement is perceived in the transverse process of the atlas. C0–C1 movement can then be assessed by introducing a springing-like motion of the head following the direction of rotation. We palpate, for example, how with left rotation the right mastoid process moves towards the ipsilateral transverse process of the atlas.

The Segmental Manual Medicine Examination

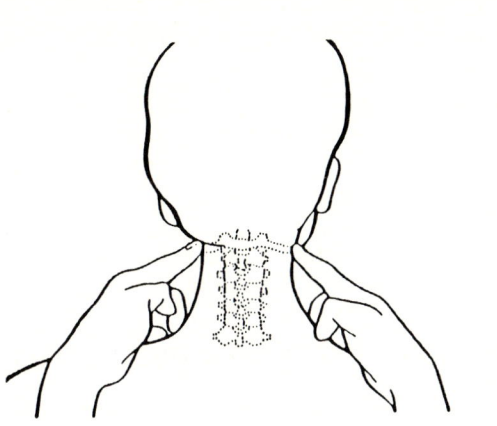

Fig. 26. Palpation of the transverse processes of the atlas with the patient seated. (After Lewit 1985)

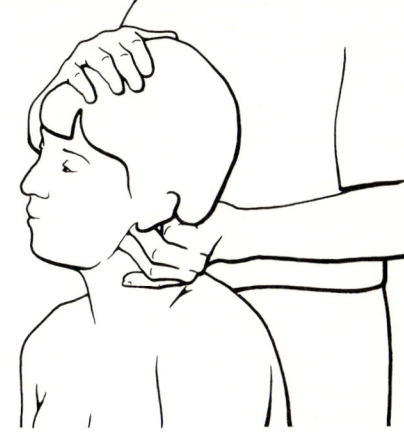

Fig. 27. Testing of the sidebending movement at the upper cervical spinal joints (C0-C1). (After Bischoff 1988)

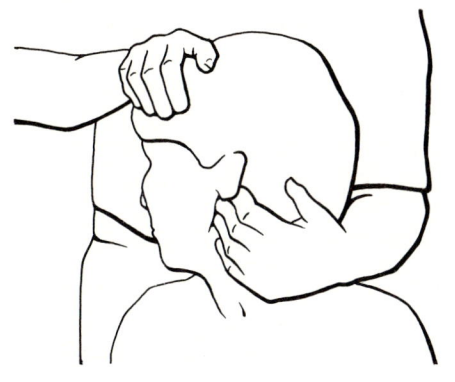

Fig. 28. Testing of the rotation movement at the upper cervical spinal joints (C0-C1). (After Bischoff 1988)

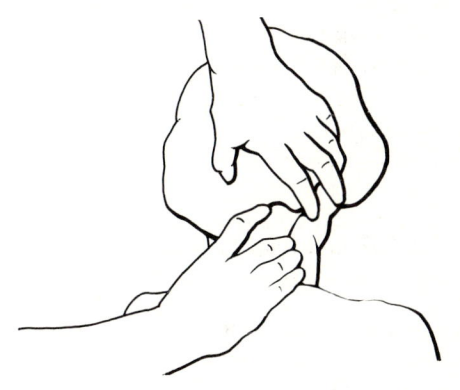

Fig. 29. Rotation motion testing at C1-C2. (After Bischoff 1988)

C1-C2:

Starting from neutral, with head rotation the spinous process of C2 does not begin to rotate until the head has rotated 20° to 30° first (Fig. 29). In the case of a somatic dysfunction, however, one can palpate how the spinous process starts to move much earlier and often immediately with the initiation of head movement.

C2-C7:

The palpating finger rests postero-laterally above the facets of the two adjoining vertebrae, with the fingertip placed over the joint space. The examiner's opposite hand guides the patient's head and cervical spine, specifically the portion superior to the spinal segment in question, into the direction that is being tested, i.e. rotation, sidebending, flexion or extension. One palpatorily evaluates the quality of joint movement and the presence of restriction along the various planes of joint movement.

The examination of the cervical spine can be performed with the patient either supine or sitting.

3.4.1.2 Thoracic Spine – Motion Testing

In practice, the first test performed is the "springing test," a maneuver that aids in saving time with localization. This test helps indicate if "something is wrong" with any of the individual segments.

The patient is prone. It is important to take out the slack and then gradually increase the pressure of the springing-like load.

Springing test – variation A: Both the index and middle finger rest over the apophyseal joints in question. The other hand lies flat over the palpating finger tips applying light pressure in a springy-type of movement (Fig. 30a, b).

Springing test – variation B: Thumb and index finger of the palpating hand grasp the spinous process of the incriminated vertebra, applying again a springy-like movement in the antero-superior direction (starting from postero-inferior, avoiding pure anterior movement).

T1–T12:

The sitting patient rests his or her shoulder against the chest of the examiner. With his free hand the examiner guides the patient's thorax into the direction that is to be evaluated. The palpating finger rests between the tips of the spinous processes of the two adjacent vertebrae. The normal findings are as follows:

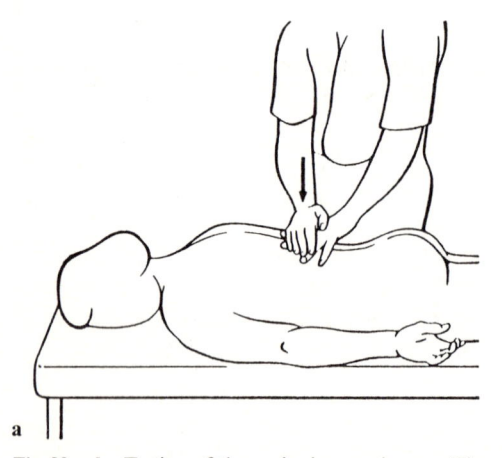

Fig. 30 a, b. Testing of the springing motion. **a** Through the ulnar border of the hand and with that arm extended the examiner introduces the springing-like force to a lumbar or thoracic vertebra. **b** Graphical representation demonstrated at a skeletal model (From Lewit 1985)

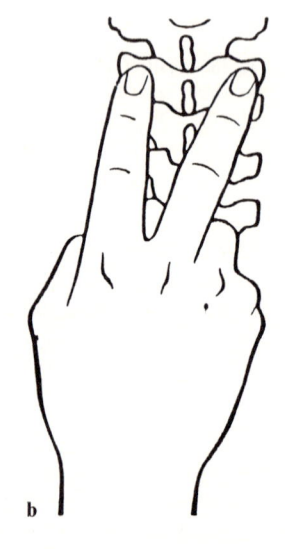

The Segmental Manual Medicine Examination 41

Rotation	– The superior spinous process of a spinal segment rotates beyond the inferior spinous process (Fig. 31).
Sidebending	– The tips of the spinous processes of the two adjoining vertebrae come together to form an angle (Fig. 32).
Flexion	– Increase in the interspinous distance (Fig. 33).
Extension	– Decrease in the interspinous distance (Fig. 34).

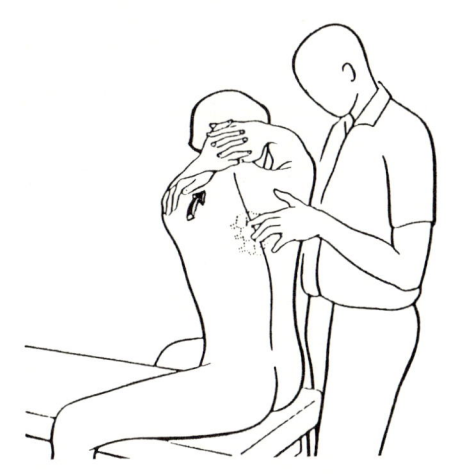

Fig. 31. Testing of the rotation movement at the thoracic spine. (From Lewit 1985)

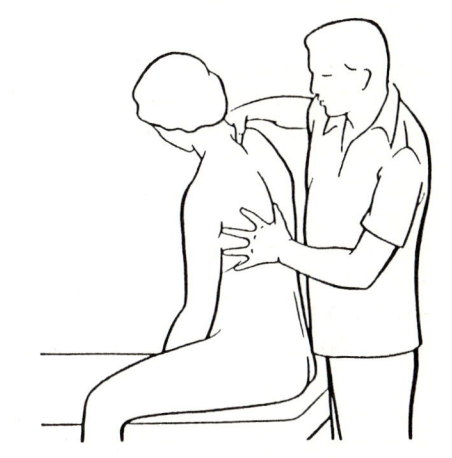

Fig. 32. Testing of the sidebending (lateral bending) movement at the thoracic spine. (From Lewit 1985)

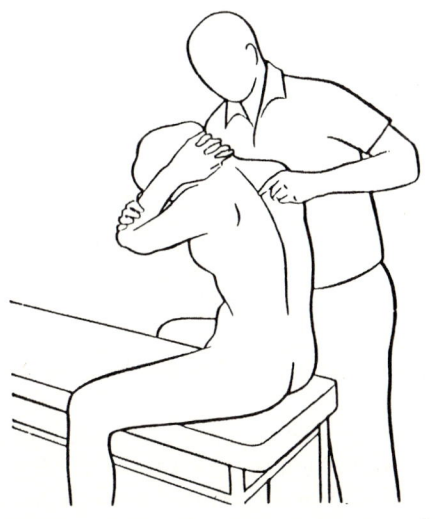

Fig. 33. Testing of the flexion movement at the thoracic spine. (From Lewit 1985)

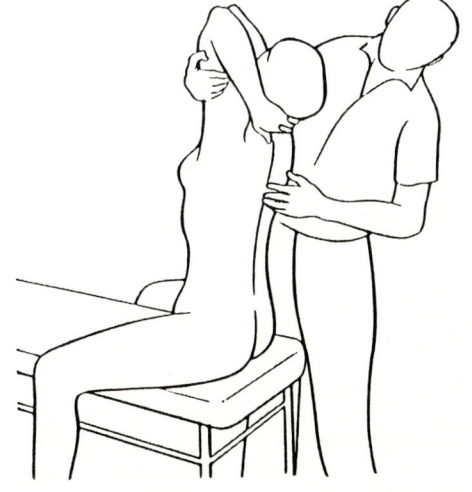

Fig. 34. Testing of the extension movement at the thoracic spine. (From Lewit 1985)

3.4.1.3 Joints Associated with the Ribs – Motion Testing

The springing test is performed with the patient prone. The thumb of the palpating hand is placed along the rib and over the intercostal space. The other hand introduces a springing-like motion to the rib in question through the palpating thumb, by moving from superior to inferior and vice versa. The shoulder blades are pulled laterally by having the patient's arms hang freely to the side.

The examination of the first rib is as follows. The patient is sitting. The head of the second metacarpal bone of the palpating hand rests between the border of the trapezius and the clavicle, beneath which is the head of the first rib. It is tested by moving it antero-medially by introducing a springing-like force tangential to the joint space.

The examination of the other ribs can be performed either with the patient sitting or supine. Some examiners prefer to have the patient supine for the entire examination while others will examine the upper five rib pairs with the patient sitting, and the lower seven pairs with the patient supine. For better control and accessibility the patient is asked to raise both of his or her arms as high as possible. For the upper five rib pairs, the palpating finger rests over the intercostal space at the level of the mamillary line, whereas for the lower seven rib pairs, the palpating finger is placed at the axillary line. The patient is requested to inhale and exhale as deeply as possible. With the patient sitting, the arm on the side that is to be examined is raised above the head so as to facilitate free breathing. When there is normally function, the intercostal space widens or narrows with inhalation and exhalation respectively. In the case of a somatic dysfunction, such respiration-dependent fluctuation will be absent. We can differentiate between an inhalation and exhalation restriction.

A somatic dysfunction affecting only one rib may, however, impair the breathing function of the entire ipsilateral hemithorax. Thus, the experienced practitioner may be able to detect visually if the hemithorax of a patient is "stuck," especially when the patient takes in a deep breath (Lewit 1977; Greenman 1979b).

3.4.1.4 Lumbar Spine – Motion Testing

The springing test is performed with the patient prone. The thenar and hypothenar eminence of the palpating hand are placed over either facet joint of the segment in question. A springing-like force is introduced through the examiner's shoulders with the elbows extended.

L1–L5

The patient is lying on his side. The palpating finger rests between the spinous processes of two adjoining vertebrae.

Rotation testing: The foot of the leg distal to the table (upper leg) is placed behind the poplitea of the lower leg, by introducing flexion to both hip and knee of the upper leg. With his free hand, the examiner rotates the pelvis so far as to engage the spinal segment in question. The next step is to palpate whether the inferior spinous process rotates further than the superior spinous process (Fig. 35).

The Segmental Manual Medicine Examination

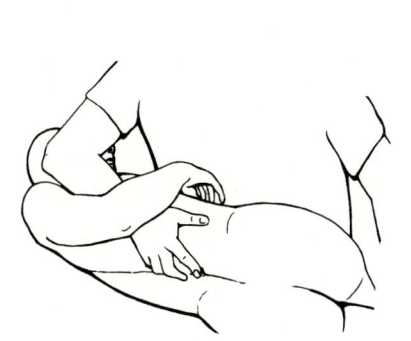

Fig. 35. Segmental rotation testing at the lumbar spine

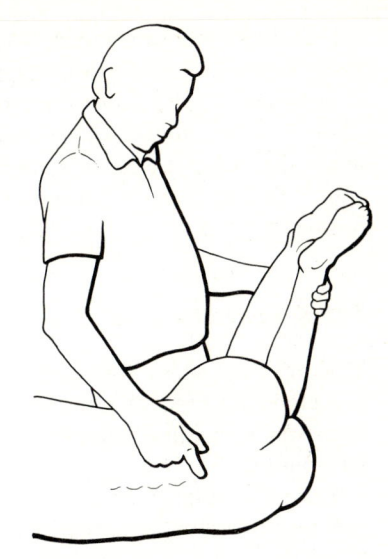

Fig. 36. Segmental sidebending (lateral bending) motion testing at the lumbar spine. (After Eder and Tilscher 1988)

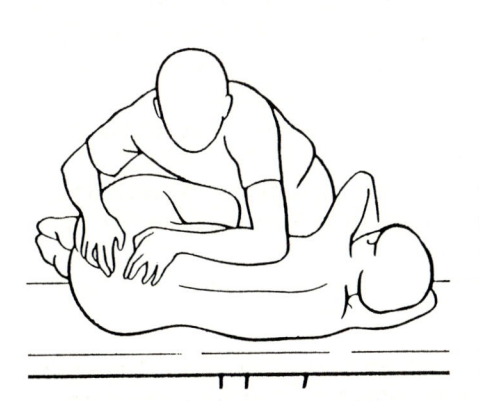

Fig. 37. Testing of the flexion movement in a lumbar spine segment. (From Lewit 1985)

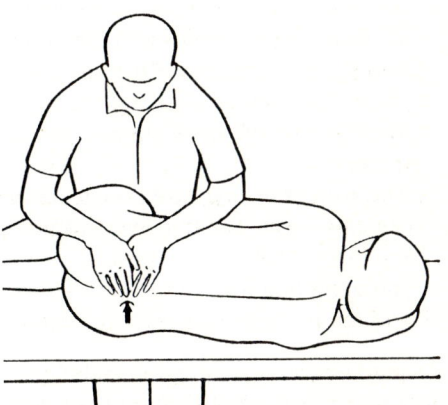

Fig. 38. Testing of the extension movement in a lumbar spine segment. (From Lewit 1985)

Sidebending testing: Both knees and hips are flexed to 90° degrees. The operator's free hand moves the patient's legs and pelvis laterally and superiorly by lifting the patient's feet at the ankles. The patient's thighs rest on the examiner's thighs. The palpating hand evaluates if any "sharp dropoffs" are present between adjoining spinous processes (Fig. 36).

Flexion testing: The patient's hips and knees are flexed. The examiner introduces flexion to the spine by flexing the patient's thighs. With the other hand he palpates the lumbar spinous processes and the interspinous distance, which normally increases with flexion (Fig. 37).

Extension testing: Both the patient's hips and knees are flexed to 90°. While stabilizing the patient's thighs with one hand, the examiner uses the other hand to guide the pelvis posteriorly thereby introducing more extension to the lumbar spine. The interspinous distance is evaluated, which should normally decrease during this procedure (Fig. 38).

3.4.1.5 Sacro-iliac Joint

Motion in the sacro-iliac joint is rather small, measuring only a few millimeters. Therefore, the functional motion testing of this joint is much more difficult than in other spinal regions. One must often perform different tests and compare the various findings.

Sacro-iliac joint function is evaluated first by utilizing the springing tests, which may be performed in various ways:

1) The patient is prone. The palpating finger rests over the sacro-iliac joint, the sacrum and the posterior superior iliac spine. The free hand introduces an anterior springing-like motion to the inferior portion of the sacrum.
2) In this variation, the patient again is prone, and the palpating finger is placed at the same location as described above. The free hand takes hold of the wing of the ilium from anterior and then rocks it back and forth. If the joint's mobility is normal, part of this rocking motion is absorbed by the joint. If, however, there is some dysfunction affecting the joint, the movement introduced to the ilium is directly transmitted to the sacrum causing it to move to the same extent as the ilium.
3) The patient in this variation is supine. The palpating finger starts out from the same position. The free hand adducts the thigh which has been flexed 90° at the hip. The thigh is then pushed in a postero-medial direction, utilizing again a springing-like force. One determines if there is movement between the sacrum and the posterior superior iliac spine.

In practice, this examination technique is often not adequate as this springing-like motion can vary significantly from patient to patient. A more reliable assessment of sacroiliac joint function can be obtained by utilizing the so called standing or seated *flexion test* (Fig. 39).

As the words imply, this test can be performed with the patient either standing or sitting. One will obtain more precise and specific information about the sacro-iliac joint itself with the patient sitting, as in the sitting position the effects of the hamstring muscles are eliminated (i.e. unilateral shortening). The patient should sit on a firm chair with the soles of the feet flat on the floor. If there is a somatic dysfunction of the sacro-iliac joint, one will observe diminished or even absent motion in that joint. The examiner palpates the most inferior portion of the posterior superior iliac spine on either side. The patient is then requested to bend forward. The examiner evaluates whether both spines move superiorly in a symmetrical fashion, or if one side moves more superiorly and anteriorly than the other.

Fig. 39. The seated flexion examination. In this example, the left side is restricted as it moves more superiorly. (After Maigne 1961)

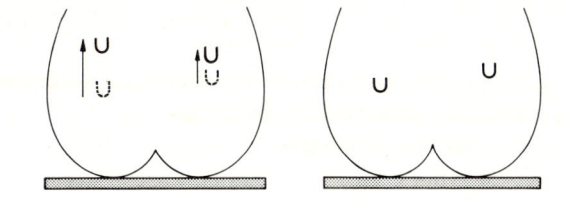

A positive seated flexion test, that is one spine moves more superiorly and anteriorly, indicates that there is a somatic dysfunction present in the ipsilateral sacro-iliac joint.

The flexion test can also be performed with the patient in a supine position. The knee joint can be either extended or flexed (elimination of the thigh extensors). First, the supine patient is instructed to sit up three times so as to balance on the ischial tuberosity. If function of sacro-iliac joint motion is impaired on one side, there will more often than not be a leg length difference.

For the purpose of differential diagnosis, one must exclude the presence of reflexive pelvic torsion. If this phenomenon is present, the flexion test is at first positive but then becomes negative after approximately twenty seconds, as in actuality there is no sacro-iliac joint dysfunction. Reflexive pelvic torsion is thought to be due to an imbalance in muscle tone, which actually may be related to dysfunctions in the upper cervical spinal joints, and occasionally the segments of L1 or L2 (Gutmann 1968).

A clear description of sacro-iliac assessment and treatment is given by Bourdillon and Day (1987).

3.4.2 Palpatory Assessment of Localized Segmental Irritation

Somatic dysfunctions affecting the facet joints are usually associated with tissue changes around the involved joint (see p. 36). These have become known as segmental irritation points, and which can be palpated as pea-sized tissue changes in the deep autochthonous muscles.

3.4.2.1 Cervical Spine

C0–C7

Patient positioning: either sitting on the examination table or supine. Examiner positioning: standing in front of the sitting patient, or seated behind the supine patient's head. The head of the seated patient's head rests comfortably against the examiner's chest. When the patient is supine, his head is held in the neutral position while it is being supported beyond the examination table on the examiner's thighs.

"Neutral position" means that, with the patient sitting, an imaginary line between the surface of the upper premolars and the mastoid process lies in the horizontal plane. With the patient supine, this line should be vertical. One should always make sure that the neutral position is maintained during the examination, as flexion and extension may either amplify or diminish the actual palpatory findings.

The local segmental zone of irritation over the joint's facets is palpated with the index or middle finger approaching the zone from posterior and through the superficial muscle layer. The next step involves the same criteria described above (Figs. 40–43). The zone of irritation associated with the atlas is palpated behind the articular process of the atlas.

The Segmental Manual Medicine Examination

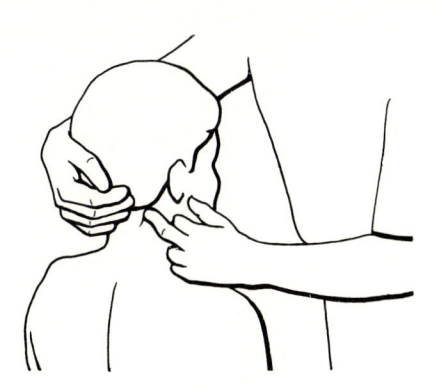

Fig. 40. Localization of the irritation point at the cervical spine. (After Bischoff 1988)

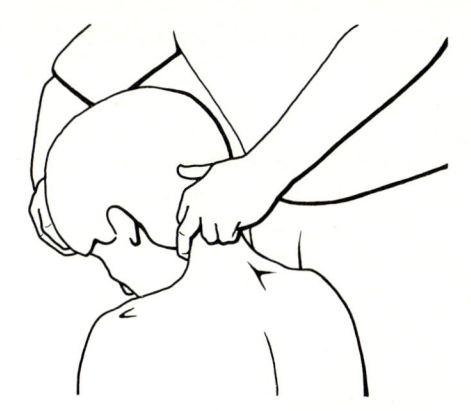

Fig. 41. Functional segmental diagnosis utilizing the irritation points at the cervical spine (during flexion testing). (After Bischoff 1988)

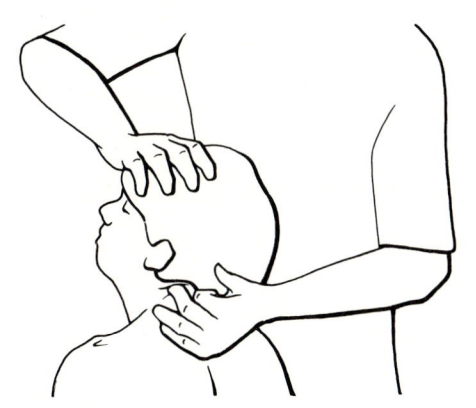

Fig. 42. Functional segmental diagnosis utilizing the irritation points at the cervical spine (during extension testing). (After Bischoff 1988)

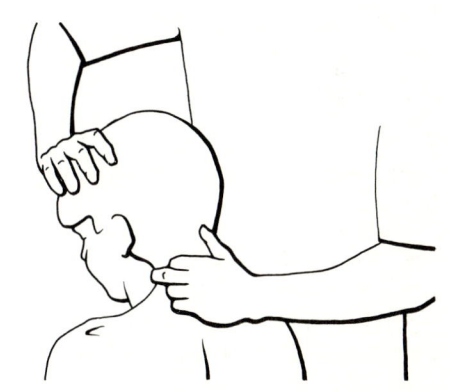

Fig. 43. Functional segmental diagnosis utilizing the irritation points at the cervical spine (during rotation testing). (After Bischoff 1988)

3.4.2.2 Thoracic and Lumbar Spine

T1-T4

Patient positioning: prone. Examiner positioning: to the side of the patient, either right or left side; either sitting or standing.

The fingertips are placed two fingerbreadths lateral to the spinous processes of the incriminated segments. Pressure is applied through the superficial muscles in the direction of the inferior facet joints (Figs. 44 and 45). Through careful layer palpation painful spasms in these muscles must be diagnostically excluded first. The muscles encountered at the T3 and T4 levels are the rhomboid muscles, while at the T1 and T2 levels it is the trapezius muscle.

T5-T9

Patient positioning: prone. Examiner positioning: standing or sitting, to the right or left of the patient.

Starting one fingerbreadth lateral to either angle of the rib each fingertip applies minimal pressure so as to push the longissimus dorsi muscle and the iliocostalis thoracis muscle towards the intercostal space. The rib is used as a guide. Once in this position, it is best to stand up and increase the anterior pressure. Starting from this, the deepest point in the intercostal space, the examiner repeats pressure in the medial direction. Thus the movement of the fingertips follow a Z- or step-like movement.

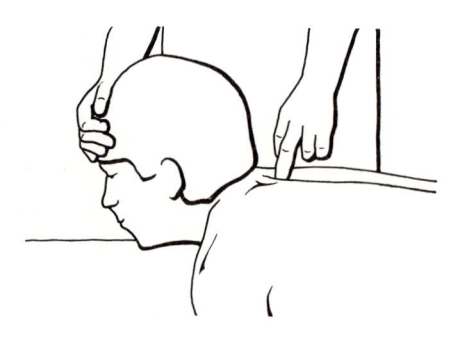

Fig. 44. Testing of irritation point during extension movement in the upper thoracic spine. (After Bischoff 1988)

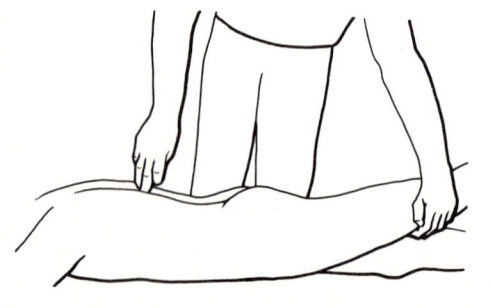

Fig. 45. Testing of irritation point during extension movement at the mid- and lower thoracic spine. (After Bischoff 1988)

The Segmental Manual Medicine Examination

T10–L1

Patient positioning: prone. Examiner positioning: sitting to the right or left of the patient.

The fingertips, which are hyperextended at the distal interphalangeal joint and placed at the lateral margin of the trunk extensor muscles, exert steady pressure in an oblique, transverse direction towards the incriminated spinal segment (Fig. 46–49). Because of the rib's resiliency in this portion of the spine, one should not utilize the rib as a guide.

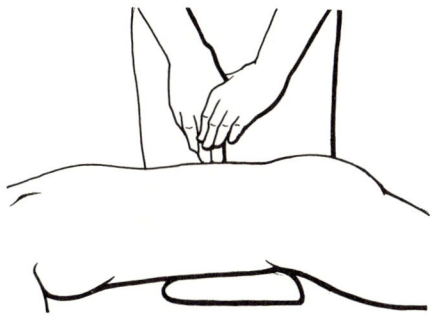

Fig. 46. Testing of the segmental irritation point by introducing flexion to the spine. (After Bischoff 1988)

Fig. 47. Testing of the segmental irritation point by introducing extension to the spine. (After Bischoff 1988)

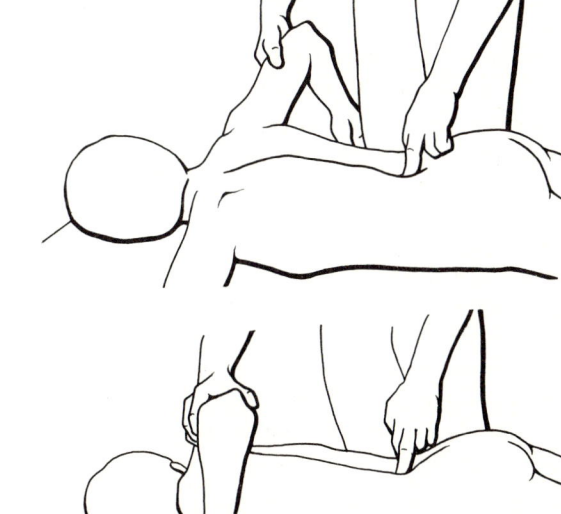

Fig. 48. Testing of the segmental irritation point at the lumbar spine by introducing rotation to the right. (After Bischoff 1988)

Fig. 49. Testing of the segmental irritation point at the lumbar spine by introducing rotation to the left. (After Bischoff 1988)

L2-L4

Patient and examiner positioning are the same as for L1.

The segmental irritation point associated with the lumbar spine can be found directly below the transverse process, approximately one fingerbreadth from the spinous process in the space formed by the row of the spinous processes and the trunk extensor muscles.

L5

Patient positioning: prone or astride the examination table. Examiner positioning: standing at the side of the patient or sitting behind her/him.

Through the hyperextended fingertips placed 1-1½ fingerbreadths above the tip of the L5 spinous process and two fingerbreadths lateral to the spinous process, one applies pressure obliquely downward in the direction of the small apophyseal joints. Pressure may be applied to both joints simultaneously or to either joint individually in an alternating fashion. After having determined the location at which there is greatest induration and tenderness, the examiner keeps steady pressure on that point, while with the other free hand, he or she passively rotates the patient's trunk into either direction so as to obtain further information for the functional diagnosis. Any active movement provided by the patient should be avoided.

3.4.2.3 Costotransverse Joints

Patient positioning: prone. Examiner positioning: sitting at either side of the patient.

The irritation points associated with the costotransverse joints are located approximately two fingerbreadths lateral to the row of the spinous processes.

The irritation points associated with the second to fourth ribs can be palpated directly posteriorly, two fingerbreadths lateral to the paraspinal muscles (Fig. 50). Pain due to the trunk extensor muscles is normally not found at this location and is therefore not expected to interfere with the diagnosis of a somatic dysfunction in this area.

The irritation point associated with the first rib can be palpated from superior by placing the tip of the middle finger over the first rib and then following it medially to the joint space.

The irritation points associated with ribs V to XI are palpated with the tip of the middle finger. Starting from the rib's angle the palpating fingertip moves along the rib in the direction of the spine, pushing beneath the trunk extensor muscles and coming as close in contact with the costotransverse joints as possible.

If there is a point of irritation, it can be further evaluated by its reaction to either inhalation or exhalation.

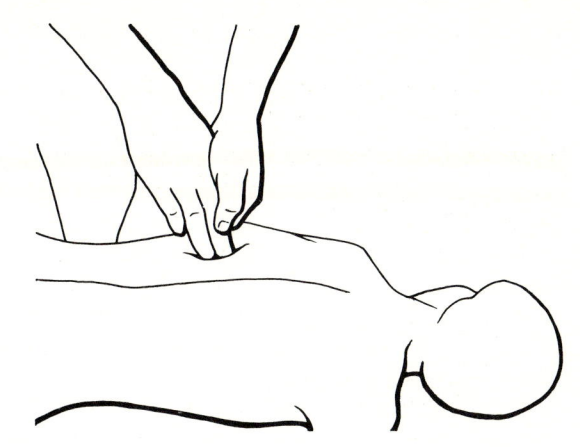

Fig. 50. Localization of the irritation point at the costotransverse joint. (After Bischoff 1988)

3.4.2.4 Sacro-iliac Joint

Patient positioning: prone. Examiner positioning: standing at the foot of the examination table.

Inspection reveals that the gluteus maximus muscle is rather flat on the side of the dysfunction. The zone of irritation for S1 is found three fingerbreadths lateral to the upper pole of the joint and four fingerbreadths inferior to the posterior superior iliac spine. The S3 zone of irritation is one fingerbreadth lateral to the lower joint pole.

One may sometimes palpate muscle spasm in the tensor fasciae latae muscle on the side opposite that where the dysfunction is thought to be.

A *dysfunction* of the sacro-iliac joint not only causes contractions and spasms in the gluteal and tensor fasciae latae muscles but may also affect the hip extensor muscles as well as the adductors. This type of finding aids in making the diagnosis of sacro-iliac joint dysfunction. The following points must be considered:

With a so called *pseudo-Lasègue* finding, the patient will complain of pain on the thigh's extensor surface down to the poplitea which worsens when the leg is raised. In contrast to a truly positive Lasègue test, where the pain comes on suddenly, there is a gradual pain increase with the pseudo-Lasègue. Motor loss is also absent and the reflexes are within the normal range (p. 98).

In order to evaluate the *abductor phenomenon* the patient must be supine. With the hip maximally abducted, the foot of the leg to be examined is placed at the medial side of the opposite knee. In the presence of a sacro-iliac joint dysfunction abduction is often (but not always!) diminished secondary to the contraction of the adductors. One must naturally exclude disorders affecting the hip, as in many instances there is abduction restriction present as well.

Quite frequently, the iliac muscle can be palpated as a painful lumpy swelling on the undersurface of the ala of the ilium, on the same side as the joint dysfunction. This *iliac swelling* may cause lower abdominal symptoms and simulate irritation of the appendix or disease of the ovaries.

In summary, segmental motion testing and segmental irritation localization are the two main diagnostic techniques used in the workup of a somatic joint dysfunction. The three-step approach summarized above (p. 35) is of great value.

3.4.3 Palpatory Assessment of Peripheral Segmental Irritation

Peripheral segmental irritation is relatively easy to localize, even if the person performing the examination has not undergone formal training in manual medicine. A prerequisite to the adequate examination, however, is that one know the dermatome supplied by the individual *ventral* ramus of the spinal nerve. With reversible somatic dysfunctions affecting a facet joint one finds skin changes, i.e. thickening of the skin (not unlike that of the so called "orange-peel" skin) and hyperalgesia in the area related to that particular spinal segment. Peripheral segmental irritation zones can be elicited by using a dermatome needle or the skin-rolling test.

Thus, a positive skin-rolling test at the eyebrow may indicate that the headache about which the patient complains is related to a dysfunction associated with the upper cervical spinal joint (leCorre 1979). This method may also be of help in the workup of nonspecific pain of the chestwall, abdomen, groin and extremities, as sometimes a somatic dysfunction can be "rolled out" (Fig. 51).

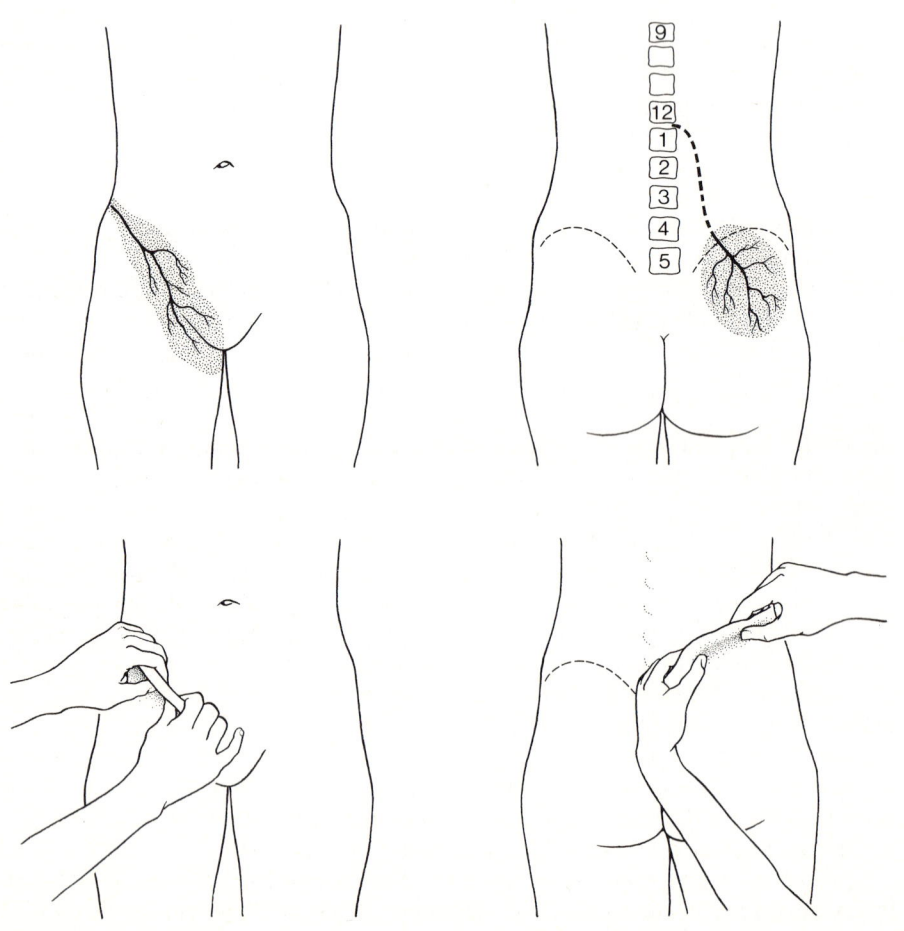

Fig. 51. Peripheral segmental irritation as demonstrated at the T12/L1 level. (After Maigne 1961)

The finding of a peripheral segmental irritation points towards the presence of a segmental joint dysfunction. The type and direction of the dysfunction can only be determined by examination of the local segmental irritation or by examination of the segmental mobility.

If the appropriate treatment to correct a reversible segmental dysfunction has been given, there is often immediate amelioration of the patient's pain in the respective dermatome, a finding which can be utilized as one indicator of the therapeutic success.

Earlier we mentioned the so called "identification" muscles (also known as "indicator" muscles, see p. 11). Thus, one would associate the presence of a radial epicondylitis with a dysfunction at the C6 level. The so called "muscle-chains" described by Bruegger (1977) deserve mentioning.

3.5 X-Ray Examination of the Spine

In Europe, Gutmann has extensively investigated how the radiological evaluation of the spine can be applied to and used in the field of manual medicine. Based on the works of Palmer (1933) and Sandberg (1955), he established basic rules for technique and interpretation of functional X-rays of the cervical and lumbar spine, pelvis and hip. The radiological evaluation of the spine is an integral part of the overall diagnostic workup.

The major tasks include:
a) to determine if there are any contraindications to using manual medicine techniques (i.e. inflammatory or destructive processes, trauma, fractures, etc.),
b) to evaluate spinal function with the patient in various positions, e.g. sitting, standing, supine.

It should be emphasized that the X-ray in and of itself does not produce the diagnosis of "somatic dysfunction." The treatment success of a manipulative procedure cannot be demonstrated via X-rays, except in rare and specific cases, as suggested by Arlen (1979).

In addition to movement, the spine has three further functions, namely those of posture, load-carrying capacity, and protection for the nerves, muscles and viscera (Kuhlendal 1970 – "the neurosymbiosis of the spine"). These three functions can be objectively and reproducibly evaluated using radiological techniques. Naturally, the X-ray examination can only be of value if it is performed accurately and consistently in a standard way (Gutmann 1975a).

The X-ray examination:
a) provides a radiological image of the individual in the neutral ("resting") position;
b) shows the individual's posture and changes when dynamic factors come into play, such as gravity, muscle pull, external loading forces;
c) provides reproducible findings ("hard copy") and thus allows comparison;
d) provides findings that can be analyzed and objectively interpreted and/or related to other findings.

3.5.1 Radiographic Technique

An X-ray of the entire spine with the patient standing would be optimal. If such a study is impossible, one should at least obtain the following two views:

1) cervical spine using the Sandberg technique,
2) lumbar spine and pelvis using the Gutmann technique.

The principles of the radiographic technique include:
a) always starting with the spine in the same initial position (i.e. sitting, standing or supine),
b) head orientation.

Cervical Spine (Antero-posterior)

(Film size: 18 × 24 cm)

The patient sits on the X-ray table. The longitudinal fold of the buttocks and the medial malleoli of both legs are in the midline of the table. The patient is asked to lie down and sit up three times, enabling her/him to come to rest on the ischial tuberosities. The head may be in a position other than the anatomical neutral position. The head position and the associated rotation should not be corrected. The upper lip and the forehead lie in one plane parallel to the table (Fig. 52).

The center of the X-ray beam is directed 1 cm inferior to both the premolars and external occiputal protuberance. The distance between the X-ray and patient is 1.5 meters. If correction of the beam direction is necessary one may simply stretch a string from the X-ray tube to the occipital protuberance and then adjust the beam along this line. This eliminates the need for a specific angle measurement.

The antero-posterior view is optimal when
- the nasal septum, the upper and lower incisors, the dens of the atlas and the body of C7 all lie in one plane,
- the mastoid processes overlap the rami of the mandible in a symmetrical fashion.

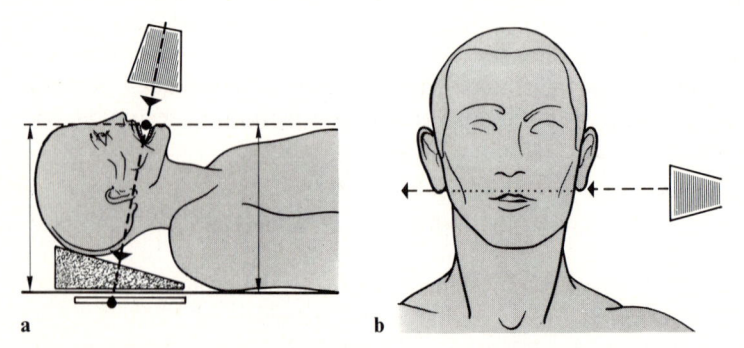

Fig. 52 a, b. X-ray technique for the cervical spine (after Gutmann). **a** Antero-posterior view (transoral view). The root of the nose and lips should lie in a line prallel to the film. **b** Lateral view: the patient is sitting. The center of the beam is directed towards the patient's earlobe

Cervical Spine (Lateral View)

(Film size 18 × 24 cm, upright)

The patient sits unsupported in front of the upright bucky, with the eyes level. The head may be repositioned only in direction of rotation and/or sidebending. The center of the beam is directed towards the earlobes, positioned at a level that divides the X-ray plate into an upper ⅓ and a lower ⅔.

The lateral view is optimal when:
- both angles of the mandible are congruent,
- the sella turcica, the hard palate and T1 are all visible,
- the hard palate is horizontal.

Lumbar Spine and Pelvis

(Film size: 30 × 40 cm, upright)

The patient stands with her/his back against the bucky. For the interpretation of this view one must assess the relationship between the so called "basic plumb-line" and the "head plumb-line" (Fig. 53). It is important that the floor be level.

The basic plumb-line is the line that falls in a plane along the midline of the X-ray plate. For practical purposes, this line may be constructed as follows: following the plate's midline down to the floor one can draw the elongation of this line on the level floor. The patient places his/her feet equidistant on either side of this line.

The head plumb-line is constructed by dropping a weight suspended from a lead string from the external occipital protuberance. This line will then show up as a marker on the X-ray plate.

The center of the beam is directed towards the iliac crest.

The lumbar spine and pelvis series are optimal when:
- T12, both femoral heads and the symphysis pubis are visualized,
- the basic and head plumb-lines are congruent.

Lumbar Spine and Pelvis (Lateral View)

(Film size: 20 × 40 cm)

The patient stands sideways with his/her left side close to the bucky. The arms are crossed in front, and the hands rest on the shoulders, providing an unobstructed view of the spine.

The basic plumb-line is erected at a distance of 3.5–4 cm from the lateral malleolus or 1 cm from the medial malleolus.

The head plumb-line (using again a lead string or wire) is erected from the external auditory foramen or the ear lobe.

The center of the beam is directed between the iliac crest and the trochanter at a level between the upper ⅔ and lower ⅓ of the X-ray plate.

The lateral lumbar spine and pelvis series is optimal when:
- T12 and the entire sacrum can be visualized.

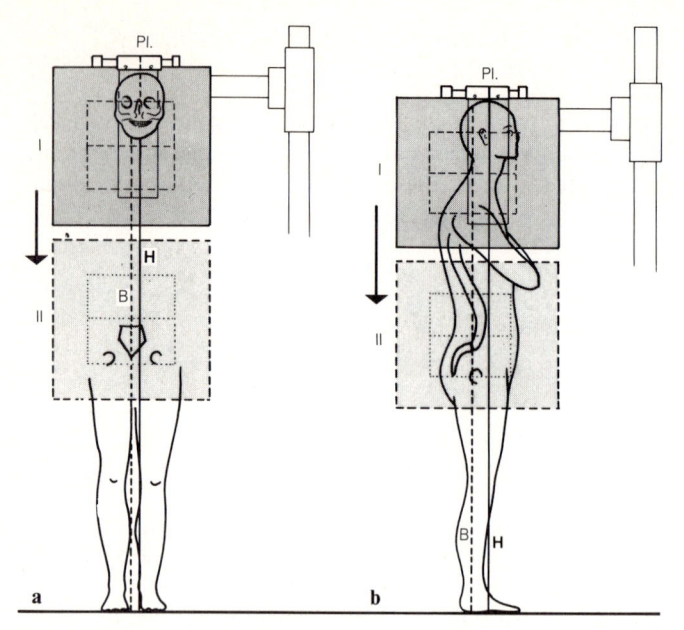

Fig. 53 a, b. X-ray technique for the lumbar-pelvic-hip region showing all the static relationships. **a** B = basic plumb-line; central line exactly between the feet (center of the filmplate as well). H = head plumb-line; plumb-line constructed through the center of gravity of the head (directed towards the center of the occipital region – external occipital protuberance). PL = moveable plexiglass attachment with connected lead string (which can according to the patient be placed over the occipital region). This attachment, once centered correctly (head plumb-line) can be lowered over the patient's lumbar-pelvic-hip region (i.e. moved from position I to position II). **b** Similar procedure for the lateral view. Here, the head plumb-line is centered at the external auditory canal, just in front of the ear lobe. Feet placement is such that the basic plumb-line is approximately one centimeter anterior to the center of the lateral malleolus The basic plumb-line is congruent with the midline of the film. Position of the head is always same: straight forward with the jaw horizontal. (After Gutmann)

3.5.2 Normal Radiographic Findings

The guidelines presented here can only serve as a mere introduction to the functional radiographic techniques and their diagnostic application in manual medicine.

A precise evaluation of the X-rays requires the use of a ruler, protractor and compass. The values reported by Gutmann (1982) are useful as a reference.

Cervical Spine (Antero-posterior)

The major landmarks are the condyles. The distance between the lateral mass and the dens of the atlas need not be interpreted at this point.

Keeping morphological and anatomical variations in mind, the following parameters are usually evaluated:

- The occipital condyles and the lower margin of the atlas run parallel.

- The condyle and atlas joint surfaces are of the same shape and length.
- The length and angle of inclination of the atlas-axis joint surfaces are symmetrical.
- The central border of the vertebral arch is perpendicular to the lateral margin of the greater occipital foramen.
- The costotransverse foramen can be visualized at either side of the axis.

Cervical Spine (Lateral)

- The tip of the dens of the atlas should be beneath the clivus of the occipital bone.
- The tip of the dens should not extend beyond the McGregor line by more than 2 cm. If the measured value is greater than 2 cm, one deals with a basilar impression (the McGregor lines runs between the lower ridge of the hard palate and the squamous portion of the occipital bone).
- The joint surfaces of the dens and the anterior arch of the atlas run parallel.
- The posterior arch of the atlas lies at the center between the occiput and C2.
- Both the anterior and posterior arch of the vertebral bodies form a smooth curve.
- The external auditory canal should not lie in front of the anterior border of the body of C7.

Lumbar Spine and Pelvis (Antero-posterior)

- The head plumb-line is congruent with the midline of the film plate.
- The femoral head and iliac crest lie in the horizontal plane.

Lumbar Spine and Pelvis (Lateral)

- The head plumb-line is congruent with the midline of the film plate.
- The contours of the hip are congruent.
- The thoracolumbar junction is posterior to the lumbosacral junction.

It would be beyond the scope of this short text to describe all the pathological findings. In reference, one may consult Gutmann's text on "Functional Pathology and Clinical Aspects of the Spinal Column" (1982).

Of interest is also the short manual by Arlen (1979) with the title "Biometric Functional X-Ray Diagnosis of the Cervical Spine." With his technique one is able to objectively document hypomobility and hypermobility of cervical spine motion in the sagittal plane (both are in German only).

3.6 Examination of Extremity Joints

Similar to the examination at the spine one proceeds from inspection to palpation to active and passive motion testing. Certain laboratory and radiographic studies may become necessary as judged by the examining physician.

Specifically, the manual examination of the extremity joints, in addition to a routine neuro-orthopedic evaluation, concentrates on the following entities:
- joint play (p. 30),
- capsular pattern (p. 58),
- muscular balance (p. 59).

Joint Play

With the joint in the neutral position, the elasticity of the ligamentous apparatus is evaluated by applying traction to the individual joint (p. 67).

This is followed by a palpatory assessment of translatory movement in a direction parallel to the various planes in a joint. At the same time joint play is evaluated. Good knowledge of the type of joint, the axes of motion and range of motion in each individual joint is indispensable. Due to the individual variation in the range of motion, one may need to examine the opposite healthy side so as to allow comparison.

In the healthy joint, palpatory perception is that of soft end-feel at the extreme of a translatory motion, which, however, may be carried further by introducing a "springing-like" movement.

If there is joint restriction, the end-feel becomes hard-elastic, and often the springing-like movement is absent.

With repetitive traction and translatory movement against the pathological barrier (p. 28) one may perceive a slow and gradual giving way of the resistance. At this point then, the diagnostic manual medicine procedure has smoothly led into the therapeutic intervention process. Passive mobilization introduced in this manner is repeated until it is felt that optimal joint function has been restored.

Joint play restoration not only improves overall joint motion, but may abolish the restriction itself.

In contrast to other standard treatment techniques (see chapter 5), the practitioner of manual medicine approaches the barrier of an extremity joint in an indirect manner. He/she treats primarily the associated translatory gliding movement, which, when improved by as little as a few millimeters, may result in an increase in angular motion by several centimeters. Herein lies one of the secrets of the success of manual medicine.

Capsular Pattern

A somatic dysfunction not only affects joint play but diminishes angular movement as well (measurable in degrees). Each joint, when affected, follows a certain pattern or sequence of restriction. This has been termed by Cyriax the *capsular pattern* (1969). If examination of a joint reveals motion restriction to differ from that expected from the joint specific capsular pattern, one must suspect other causes such as trauma, inflammatory processes, loose joint bodies or causes associated with structures surrounding the joint.

The capsular pattern has been described only for those joints which are moved by muscles. Thus, there is no capsular pattern for such joints as the acromio-clavicular and sacro-iliac joints (Winkel et al. 1985).

The capsular pattern for some extremity joints is as follows:

- shoulder: abduction – external rotation – internal rotation
- elbow: flexion – extension
- wrist: equal limitation of flexion and extension
- carpometacarpal joint I: abduction and extension limitation to the same extent; nonrestricted flexion
- interphalangeal joints: flexion – extension
- hip joint: extension – internal rotation – abduction – external rotation
- knee joint: gross limitation of flexion (i.e. 90°) – slight limitation of extension (i.e. 5–10°). Rotation is limited only if there is major reduction in the flexion/extension motion
- ankle joint (subtalar): plantarflexion – dorsiflexion (if the calf muscles are not shortened)
- Talo-calcaneo-navicular joint: increasing limitation of varus until fixation in valgus
- Tarso-metatarsal joint: dorsiflexion – plantarflexion – adduction internal rotation remain unlimited
- Metatarso-phalangeal joint I: gross limitation in extension (i.e. 60–80°) – flexion (i.e. 10–20°)
- Remaining 4 MTP joints: flexion in the MPT joint, extension in the IP joints.

In most cases, restriction occurs primarily in one direction first which can easily be found in the physical examination (usually the restriction becomes unequivocally prominent). For example, at the shoulder the pattern is primarily that of limitation of abduction, followed by external rotation and, lastly, by limitation of internal rotation. Functional joint mobility is restored in the reverse order, that is, in the shoulder, the first to return is internal rotation, followed by external rotation and finally abduction. One may gauge the therapeutic success by the return of the specific movement component.

Muscular Balance

Muscle function testing, part of which is manual muscle testing, is an essential part of the specific manual examination of the joints. Even though it is important to gain an initial impression about muscle strength and function, the specific manual medicine examination at this point concentrates on evaluating muscle balance and coordination.

According to their reaction to dysfunction, the muscles can be classified in two major groups, namely the phasic and tonic (postural) muscles (Table 2).
The phasic muscles are primarily composed of fast twitch muscle fibers (type II, "white"), which tend to fatigue more easily, recover more slowly and atrophy when there is associated dysfunction. In contrast, the tonic or postural muscles (Fig. 54) are made up primarily of slow twitch fibers (type I, "red"), which fatigue less easily, recover more quickly and tend to shorten in the presence of dysfunctions.

For example, the shortening of the iliopsoas muscle and atrophy of the gluteal muscles will lead to limited extension at the hip. This is associated with an exag-

Table 2. Phasic and tonic muscles

Postural (tonic) muscles slow twitch fibers fatigue less quickly, tend to shorten	Phasic muscles fast twitch fibers fatigue quickly, tend to atrophy
Gastrocnemius muscle Soleus muscle Rectus femoris muscle Tensor fasciae latae muscle Sartorius muscle Biceps femoris muscle Semitendinosis muscle Semimembranosus muscle Short hip adductor muscles Iliopsoas muscle Piriformis muscle Back extensor muscles Quadratus lumborum muscle Pectoralis major muscle (sternal portion) Sternocleidomastoid muscle Upper trapezius muscle Scalene muscles Levator scapulae muscle Hand flexor muscles	Anterior tibialis muscle Vastus lateralis muscle Vastus medialis muscle Gluteus maximus muscle Long hip adductor muscles Gluteus medius muscle Abdominal muscles Rhomboid muscles Serratus anterior muscle Middle and lower trapezius muscle Intrinsic muscles of the hand and foot

geration of the lumbar lordosis which in turn can lead to other somatic dysfunctions in more distant areas of the spine.

Shortening of the pectoralis major muscle restricts elevation of the shoulder. As the rhomboid muscles are frequently weak it is easy to see that one can develop chronic shoulder, neck and arm pain. Both of these examples have deliberately been kept simple. Quite frequently, entire chains of muscles are affected requiring a profound knowledge of anatomy and a logical, well organized examination routine (Fig. 55).

Janda (1976) presents an approach for length testing of the tonic muscles and for strength testing of the phasic muscles.

One of the possible explanations for muscular imbalance may be the poor adaptation of the musculo-skeletal system to modern day activities, as too much sitting, abnormal posture at work and inappropriate athletic training are quite the rule. In daily clinical practice, it is one of the major causes for chronic complaints, not only in the extremities but also, and perhaps more importantly, in the shoulder-neck and lumbar-pelvis regions. Even in children muscular imbalance has frequently been observed.

Joint disturbances can lead to muscular imbalance and vice versa. Either abnormality must be accurately recognized, and the significance of its contribution to the overall disturbance must be assessed.

The ultimate goal of the diagnosis and treatment in manual medicine is the restoration of function in the musculoskeletal system.

Examination of Extremity Joints

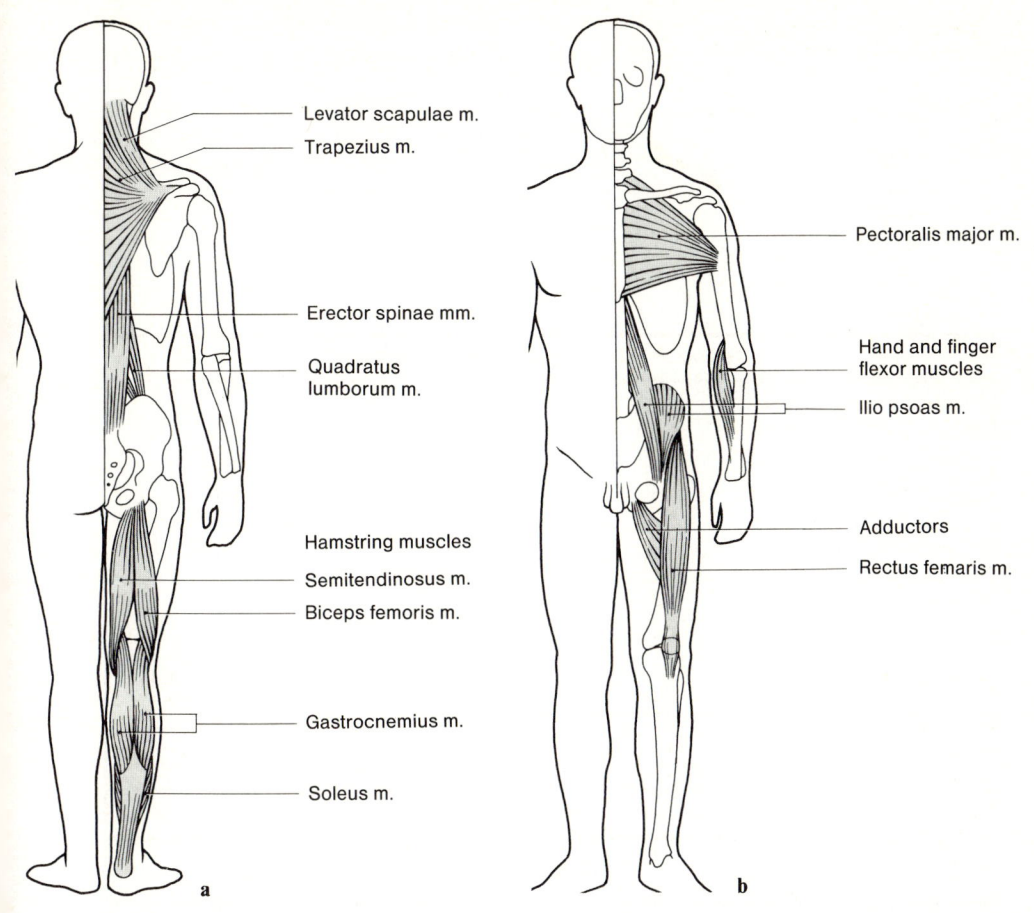

Fig. 54. Tonic muscles which are often shortened. (After Janda 1970)

Fig. 55. a Muscular balance. *1*, neck extensor muscles; *1a*, neck flexor muscles; *2*, thorax extensor muscles; *3*, Lumbar extensor muscles; *3a*, abdominal flexor muscles. **b** Muscular imbalance. 1/2/3, Increased tone (tension in the extensor musculature); *1a/3a*, weak flexor muscles. (From Huguenin 1985)

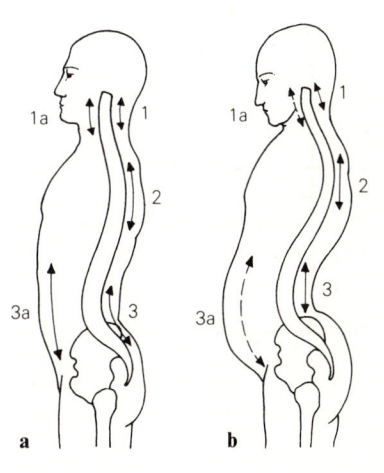

4 Manual Therapy

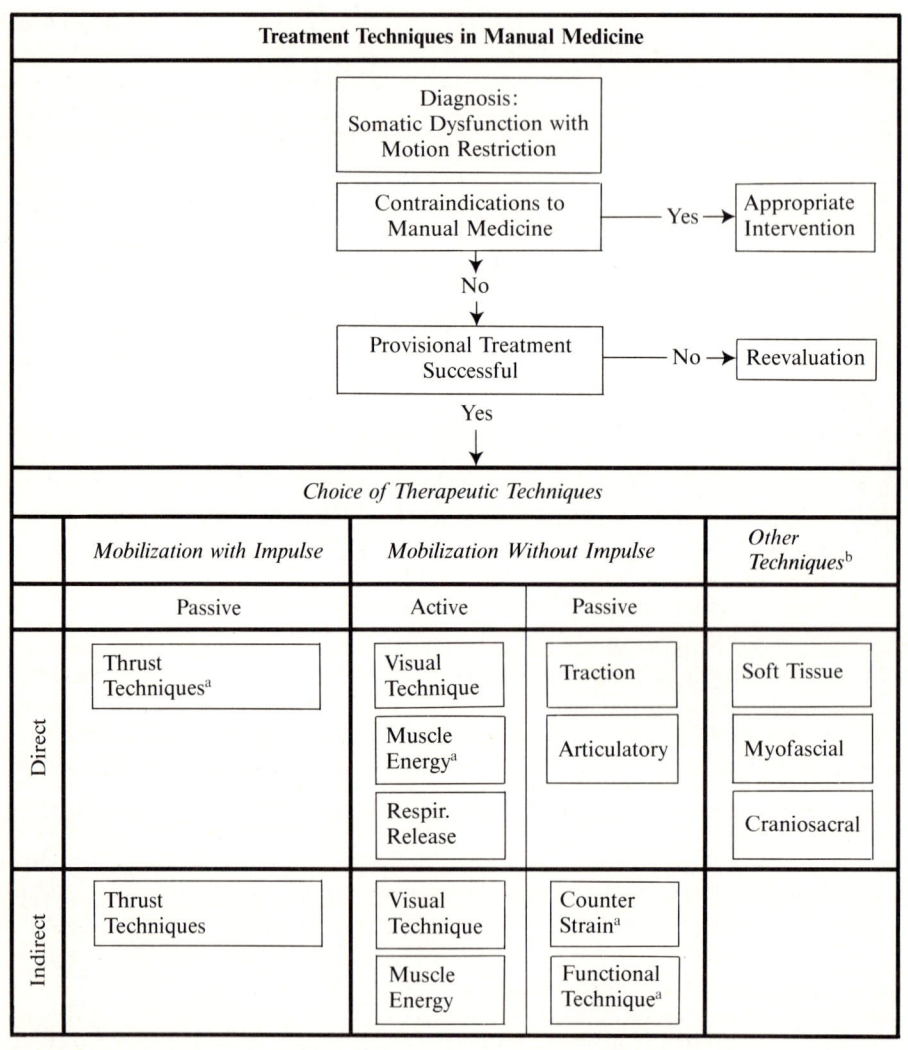

Treatment Techniques in Manual Medicine				
	Diagnosis: Somatic Dysfunction with Motion Restriction → Contraindications to Manual Medicine — Yes → Appropriate Intervention; No ↓ Provisional Treatment Successful — No → Reevaluation; Yes ↓
	*Choice of Therapeutic Techniques*
	Mobilization with Impulse		*Mobilization Without Impulse*	*Other Techniques*[b]
	Passive	Active	Passive	
Direct	Thrust Techniques[a]	Visual Technique / Muscle Energy[a] / Respir. Release	Traction / Articulatory	Soft Tissue / Myofascial / Craniosacral
Indirect	Thrust Techniques	Visual Technique / Muscle Energy	Counter Strain[a] / Functional Technique[a]	

[a] Indicates in which category (direct vs. indirect) the technique is usually applied.
[b] Please note that the "Other Techniques" are not clearly divided into direct vs. indirect techniques.

Manual Therapy

The goal of the various manual therapy techniques is to bring about recovery or amelioration of reversible functional disturbances (somatic dysfunctions), at either the spine or an extremity joint or both.

Successful treatment requires good cooperation between patient, physician and physical therapist. The physician makes the diagnosis, formulates the therapeutic approach and performs the treatment procedure, especially such techniques as manipulation with impulse and the classical low-amplitude, high-velocity thrust techniques.

The appropriately trained physical therapist is able to apply certain soft tissue and/or mobilization techniques. In recent years, the scope of a physical therapist's expertise has considerably increased, especially with the advent of such techniques as muscle inhibition and facilitation.

Incorrect posture and muscle imbalance has become one of the most frequent causes of joint dysfunctions. In order to improve the patient's dysfunctions the underlying cause must be determined if possible. If postural or muscle imbalance plays a significant role, needs to be addressed right from the start with appropriate changes such as assuming correct posture at the workplace and altering faulty movements during the performance of the daily living activities. In addition, the patient must properly learn a specific set of exercises that he/she will perform on a regular basis (e.g. "back school").

The cooperative interplay between patient, physician and physical therapist makes this a true *team* approach with the goal being a patient's complete and successful rehabilitation.

> The classical thrust techniques, also known as "mobilization with impulse" techniques, should only be performed by licensed personnel. It must be emphasized that prior to the application of this technique any contraindications must be excluded.

Manual therapy is certainly not a "bump and crack" method. It resorts to a set of different techniques which are used in response to the individual diagnostic findings. It is beyond the scope of this introductory text to describe all of the various techniques. For brevity and a general overview the discussion here will concentrate on those techniques most frequently encountered and used.

Classification of the different techniques is not that simple as there may be overlap between the various techniques. There are, however, basic principles of technique which are common to all procedures and should be understood by the practitioner of manual medicine. Beal's concise review (1982) of some of those underlying principles provides a clear understanding of direct versus indirect and long versus short leverage procedures, for instance. Another, more inclusive categorization is presented by Briner et al. (1981), who distinguish between primarily mechanical or neuro-reflexive approaches, focusing on bony positional changes, soft tissue changes, sensory and/or motor points, central nervous and body rhythm involvement and the body's accommodations to environmental demands.

Again, as stated earlier, the cause of a somatic dysfunction is thought to involve multivariate changes and should therefore respond to various procedures. The following classification, based on what are felt to be some of the major principles, is used to provide the reader with a general but clear introduction to the most important techniques. As pointed out by Beal (1982), critical factors in the skillful use of manipulative techniques include accurate localization and constant monitoring during the execution of each procedure.

The goal of treatment is to decrease joint restriction and the associated mechanical and reflex changes so as to restore joint function to as close to normal as possible.

Treatment can be performed by engaging the restrictive barrier either *directly* or *indirectly*. This means that the patient is moved (by the operator, passively) or he/she (actively) moves towards or away from the barrier (Fig. 56 a and b). In the indirect method the reciprocal inhibitory mechanisms are utilized. The terms "active" and "passive" will be described further in Sect. 4.2.

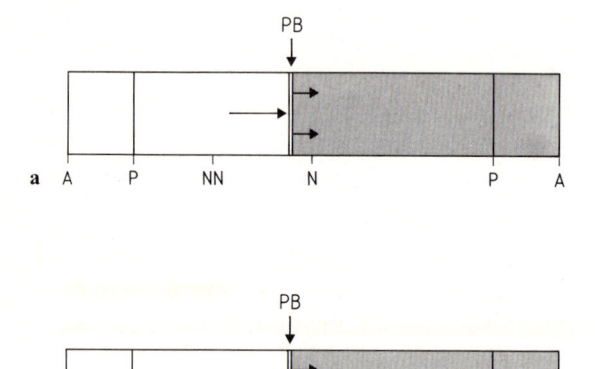

Fig. 56. **a** The direct engagement of the barrier. **b** The indirect engagement of the barrier. *PB*, pathological barrier; *A*, anatomical barrier; *P*, physiological barrier; *N*, neutral position (point); *NN*, new neutral position; *shaded area*, equal degree of motion loss

4.1 Soft Tissue Techniques

Perhaps the best and most logical way to get acquainted with some of the principles in manual therapy is via the soft tissue techniques. Mastery of these techniques provides the practitioner not only with a set of specific manual medicine maneuvers but, equally important, facilitates the development of palpatory skills, the "feel" for the tissues which is essential to the manual medicine approach.

Tight muscles associated with a restricted joint can be relaxed by transverse and longitudinal stretching techniques as can be some of the soft tissue swelling. Cyriax's "deep friction massage" is another example of a soft tissue technique. In some clinical settings certain other mobilization techniques can only be performed once the tissues have been "prepared" by the soft tissue techniques.

Soft tissue techniques may be complemented by therapeutic physical exercises, electrotherapy, skin stimulation or other appropriate physiotherapeutic measures as long as they are indicated and properly applied.

4.2 Mobilization Techniques Without Impulse

We differentiate between active and passive mobilization techniques. Active motion is that movement produced voluntarily by the patient (muscle contraction, respiration, gaze). Passive motion is that induced by the operator while the patient remains passive or relaxed (Ward 1981). A further distinction as to the type of technique is whether the restrictive barrier is engaged directly or indirectly (Fig. 55). Examples of the direct technique include the muscle energy and articulatory techniques. Representatives of the indirect technique are the functional and strain/counterstrain techniques. There is, of course, some overlap between the various types, which, at the beginning, may be the cause of some confusion. For didactical purposes, the techniques which will be decribed in the following paragraphs have been grouped according to broader classification schemes.

First, some of the principles of the passive techniques are presented, followed by a short description of the articulatory technique. Subsequently the reader is introduced to the active mobilization techniques with the muscle energy technique being the typical representative. The discussion then shifts to the description of the indirect method of treatment including the functional and strain/counterstrain techniques (both of which are passive techniques).

It is hoped that the diagram on page 62 will aid in clarifying some of the concepts, especially describing the overlap and the differences between the individual techniques as well.

4.2.1 Passive Mobilization

Starting from the joint's neutral position (resting or "present neutral" position), passive mobilization is carried out either parallel or perpendicular to the tangential plane of the incriminated joint. In the neutral position, the joint capsule is maximally relaxed and has greatest joint volume.

While one joint partner remains stationary (fixed in a controlled manner by the practitioner) the other is mobilized. The points of contact should be as close to either side of the joint space without actually coming in contact with the joint itself.

Passive mobilization begins with *traction* perpendicular to the tangential plane of the incriminated joint. According to Derbolowsky (1976) traction is introduced in a stepwise approach:

Step I – loosening,
Step II – "taking out the slack",
Step III – stretching.

Step I: Minimal traction is introduced to the joint, the force being of sufficient magnitude to just neutralize the pressure between the two joint partners but not to distract the joint surfaces.

Step II: More tractional force is introduced here to the joint along the longitudinal axis such that the "slack" is taken out. Bringing a joint into this position must be done before the joint can be stretched. Equally important, traction at this level may ameliorate the patient's pain and thus may be utilized when other techniques are not indicated because they cause pain.

Step III: The soft tissues are stretched further yet. Mobilization proceeds in smooth, rhythmic distraction movements, which are repeated 8 to 10 times. In summary, the sequence of traction using passive mobilization includes the following steps: loosening – taking out the slack – stretching to the physiological barrier – hold at the barrier – hold – hold – release (but not below level II, not to the starting neutral position), repeat if necessary, etc.

In clinical situations in which mobilization with impulse (the classic thrusting techniques) is being considered, similar preparation may be necessary before applying the actual thrusting force (i.e. impulse, p. 73).

Gliding mobilization is performed along the tangential plane of the incriminated joint. Simultaneously, traction is applied but only of sufficient strength to neutralize the pressure between the two joint partners (level II). The capsule must not be stretched as far as with the pure traction techniques as some of the gliding movement may otherwise be lost. The practitioner is then able to engage the pathological barrier he had diagnosed in his workup (joint play). If this is painful to the patient, one may try to work in the opposite, that is the pain-free, direction (Fig. 57).

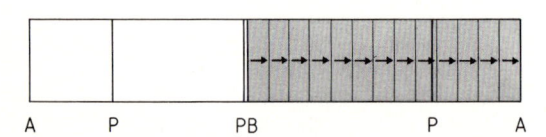

Fig. 57. Stepwise gain in range of motion by mobilization

After 8 to 10 such mobilization movements joint play and angular movement are reevaluated. If there is no noticeable movement one should reassess the diagnosis and possibly formulate a new one as well as plan the appropriate therapeutic approach.

Convex-Concave Rule (Kaltenborn 1976)

In all joints, *angular* movement in a particular direction is always associated with a rolling movement in the same direction. The associated *translatory* gliding motion direction, however, depends on the shape of the joint partner that is moving (is being moved):

1) Gliding is in the opposite direction when the moving joint surface is convex.
2) Gliding is in the same direction when the moving joint surface is concave.

Thus, the axis of movement is always localized at the convex joint partner, which in one case is the fixed and in the other the moving portion.

Thus, the practitioner must know whether the particular joint surface of the mobile joint partner is convex or concave, as the direction in which the gliding mobilization proceeds is directly related to the anatomy of the joint surface. This is demonstrated in Fig. 58.

There, in both examples, the left joint partner is fixed, while the right partner is moved. In this situation then, where the motion of the mobile joint partner is in the upward direction, one can see that

1) translatory gliding is downward with the convex surface, and
2) translatory gliding is upward with the concave surface.

Passive mobilization treatment can be given to any joint in which a reversible functional disturbance with motion restriction is present. Complications are quite rare, especially when one always keeps in mind that manual therapy is to be pain-free. In daily clinical practice, passive mobilization procedures play a major role in the treatment of restricted extremity joints. The practitioner will be continually surprised by the treatment successes seen with these techniques, especially in comparison with other physical therapeutic treatments, for instance.

4.2.1.1 Articulatory Technique

Actually, the articulatory technique as well as its close relative, the springing technique, can be viewed as an extension of the diagnostic procedures and soft tissue techniques. Using a low velocity/high amplitude approach, the barrier is repeated-

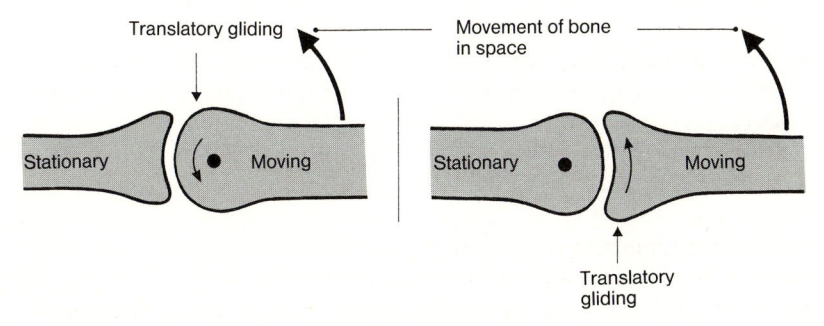

Fig. 58. The concave-convex rule. (After Kaltenborn 1976)

ly engaged (in a direct fashion), then disengaged, only to be engaged again. The goal of this technique is to bring about an increase in mobility, and if possible to restore normal range of motion.

4.2.2 Active Mobilization

Not until rather recently have the importance and effectiveness of the active mobilization techniques been realized. They are especially useful when dealing with a nervous or apprehensive patient, or if there is extreme pain or the patient demonstrates a poor general health status. In many instances, active mobilization procedures can be used in place of the passive and even some thrust (impulse) techniques. However, they are not appropriate as an alternative treatment procedure in all cases. Examples of active mobilization techniques include the muscle energy technique, visual facilitation technique, and the respiratory technique which will be decribed in more detail in the ensuing sections.

4.2.2.1 Muscle Energy Technique

The muscle energy technique (MET) was developed by F. Mitchell Sr. in the early 1960's (Mitchell et al. 1979). This is a manual medicine procedure that differs from others by the fact that the mobilization force is generated by the patient and not by the practitioner. It is of utmost importance that the restricted joint is engaged precisely at the pathological barrier and the patient is guided appropriately by the practitioner with regard to the strength and direction of the mobilization force.

MET can be applied to any movable joint. The following example utilizing joint restriction at the apophyseal joint may illustrate the basic principles.

1) Accurate diagnosis: After the restricted spinal segment has been identified, one has to further determine in which of the planes movement has become restricted (i.e. flexion-extension, sidebending, rotation).
2) Accurate patient positioning: The spinal segments above and below the incriminated segement are "locked" or fixed, that is "slack" is taken out in the neighboring segments. In this way the restricted spinal segment is specifically localized and then the joint carried to the resistant barrier along any of the three planes. Tissue changes around the joint can be used to monitor the positioning and localization (i.e. via accompanying tissue tension changes, pain perception, etc.).
   It is extremely important that the patient be carried to the barrier rather gently and smoothly, with as little jerky and abrupt movement as possible (the patient is being "nudged").
3) The patient is requested to provide an equal but opposite counterforce to that provided by the practitioner (along the three planes of motion restriction at the motion barrier).
   The following three points should always be kept in mind:
   - the force of contraction (against the resistance provided by the practitioner) is dependent on which joint is involved (50 p to 500 p); thus dosage must be individualized,

- direction of force,
- duration of contraction, i.e. force delivery time; usually around 5 seconds.

The practitioner must constantly monitor tissue changes over the incriminated area.

4) The patient is then requested to completely relax whilst remaining in this new position, that is he/she should not move actively at this time.
5) The joint then is able to undergo a mobility increase during the postisometric relaxation period, which lasts between 10 and 30 seconds (Lewit 1985). Thus, the pathological barrier approaches the physiological barrier. The practitioner subsequently guides the patient to the newly established resistant barrier, again continually monitoring tissue response. This must be done in a very gentle and careful manner, avoiding abrupt and forceful movements.
6) Steps 2-5 are repeated two or three times, depending on the patient's response to the individual treatment procedure.
7) Reevaluation and possible repetition of the entire treatment.

If this technique is painful to the patient, one may, instead of this direct technique, apply the principles of indirect techniques, that is guide the incriminated joint away from the restrictive barrier.

The inappropriate execution of the MET technique can be attributed to mistakes made by either the practitioner, the patient or both.

Major mistakes made by the practitioner:
1) forceful engagement of the pathological barrier; the barrier should be engaged in a soft, smooth manner ("nudged"),
2) direction and degree of force and counterforce are not in balance and/or inappropriate,
3) the pause between individual contraction periods is too short,
4) poor localization.

Major mistakes made on part of the patient:
1) too great a force (inappropriate dosage),
2) wrong direction,
3) too quick or jerky relaxation ("let-go") after contraction.

The entire procedure should be performed in a calm and smooth manner. Jerky, abrupt movements must be avoided by both the practitioner and patient. The principle here is to *"balance the forces,"* which requires exact positioning and localization of the joint and gentle but exact engagement at the barrier.

Lewit and Gaymans have proposed a series of selfmobilization techniques based on the MET technique (Lewit and Gaymans 1980; Lewit 1985).

The preceding description demonstrated how the MET can be used to actively mobilize a joint. Mitchell has already expanded this concept and pointed out how, in addition to disturbances arising from the joint itself, this technique can be utilized when there is loss of motion secondary to muscle involvement. If the overall function of the musculoskeletal system is to be restored, it is simply not sufficient to treat the mechanical causes arising from the joint itself. It is equally important to address and correct any coexisting muscular imbalance.

Muscular imbalance may be due to weakening of the phasic muscles on one side and shortening of the postural muscles on the other side (see page 58). The weakened muscles are strengthend through isotonic and in particular isometric exercises. The shortened muscles can be stretched through specific stretching exercises (Anderson 1982) or may be stretched during the postisometric relaxation phase (Janda 1970; Hamberg and Evjenth 1982; Lewit 1985).

According to Janda, it is important to stretch the shortened muscles before strengthening the weak muscles; in many instances, the weak muscles recover as soon as the shortened muscles had been given the opportunity to be stretched.

> Stretching comes before strengthening.

Remember: before treating a muscular problem it is important to treat the joint dysfunction and its immediate changes first.

In summary, the following considerations are important: The MET improves overall mobility in the musculoskeletal system and muscular balance by

- improving joint motion restrictions (dysfunctions),
- stretching shortened muscles,
- strengthening weak muscles.

4.2.2.2 Visual Facilitation Technique (Gaymans 1978)

Associated with each eye movement is motion at the head and spine. This can be demonstrated as follows: place the index finger of each hand on either side of the transverse process of the atlas and then move your eyes up and down, with the head stationary and the spine in neutral position. You will feel slight movement at the atlas synchronous with and in the same direction as the eye movement.

This visual facilitation technique is especially well suited for treatment of dysfunctions localized primarily at the cervical spine. Analogous to the MET technique, the joint is carried to its barrier along all three planes. One hand, the monitoring hand, fixes the vertebra below the incriminated segment and simultaneously registers any tissue change. The other hand fixes, with minimal pressure, the patient's head in a direction opposite that of the pathological barrier.

Again, an indirect method, though less frequently used, is equally applicable. The positioning of the joint at the barrier in all three planes must be done very meticulously. The monitoring hand will detect any tissue change (i.e. change of muscle tension in the long and short muscles of the back) and thus is able to determine if positioning occurred in the right direction.

The patient is now requested to change his/her gaze in a direction tangential to the plane of the restricted joint. One may use the numbers on the face of a clock as a directional guide. While the patient is looking towards the restricted side, the palpating fingers perceive an increase in tissue tension. In contrast, with the patient looking away from the restricted side one will perceive a decrease in tissue tension. Each step lasts approximately five seconds and the movement is repeated 3 or 4 times. Again, after completion of the procedure the patient is re-evaluated.

The visual facilitation technique is very gentle and may, if not successful in resolving a restriction totally, at least help in preparing and setting up the joint for other procedures such as the thrust (impulse) techniques.

4.2.2.3 Respiratory Release Technique

Muscle tone undergoes periodic changes synchronously with the respiratory movement. Thus, voluntary respiratory effort can be utilized as an additional technique in conjunction with other mobilization procedures.

The increase in tone associated with deep inhalation, for instance, may be sufficient to mobilize a joint that has been engaged accurately and properly at its restrictive barrier. Also, during the execution of the mobilization technique with impulse (thrust), the thrusting force is best introduced at the end of deep exhalation, taking advantage of the associated muscle relaxation at that moment.

In addition to changes in muscle tone, respiratory effort brings about changes in the spinal curves. During inhalation, the normal curvatures of the spine flatten, while during exhalation they become more pronounced. At the same time, the extremity joints undergo external and internal rotation, respectively, which may be used to mobilize restricted joints.

4.3 Indirect Techniques

As stated above, the indirect technique is a treatment modality in which, in contrast to the direct techniques, the motion barrier is disengaged. The lesioned complex is moved away from the motion barrier to a point of simultaneous balance and decreased tension (Ward 1981). The typical representatives are the functional and strain/counterstrain techniques, both of which are passive techniques and require good palpatory skills as well as good sense of balance in the three planes of motion.

4.3.1 Functional Technique

This therapeutic method requires an approach completely different to everything explained up to this point. In this technique, the patient is guided away from the pathological barrier so as to find a joint position of ease (Hoover 1958; Bowles 1981). The practitioner continuously monitors in the area associated with the dysfunctional segment or joint complex any physiological and non-physiological response in the tissues to the specifically introduced motion. Using his/her palpatory skills the practitioner determines the point at which localized tissue tension associated with the dysfunction is least (i.e. trigger points or zone of irritation), that is he/she guides the patient to the position of spontaneous release. The direction of this positioning is towards immediate ease and comfort; it was described by Hoover as "dynamic neutral." The concept of dynamic neutral implies seeking a bilateral balance of tension near the anatomical neutral position.

The phenomenon can be observed, for instance, when the patient guards one specific position as a result of an inflamed joint. A patient with arthritis of the hip may bring his/her affected joint into slight abduction, external rotation and flexion, the joint's present "dynamic neutral" position; the joint capsule and associated muscles, tendons and ligaments are optimally relaxed, albeit out of balance.

A restricted joint that has lost part of its mobility will also change its original (anatomical) neutral point (see Fig. 56). Consequently, there arises an imbalance in the muscles, as they undergo contraction in the direction of motion restriction. Utilizing his/her palpatory skills, the practitioner then must localize the new "neutral" or what has been called the "present neutral" (or "dynamic neutral") position of each restricted joint. This is done as follows:

The patient sits upright, with the spine in the overall neutral, that is neither flexed or extended, position. One may, however, examine the cervical and thoracic spine with the patient in the supine position. Constantly monitoring tissue changes, the operator places one hand over the area of the incriminated joint. The tissue changes associated with movement along the three planes of the restricted joint may be very subtle, and significant practice and concentration are required to detect these. Moving the patient towards the motion barrier increases the sense of tissue resistance and, conversely, guiding the patient away from the barrier decreases the sense of tissue resistance. With the help of palpation one is then able to determine where tissue tension is least in all three angular planes of the incriminated joint. This is followed by positioning the joint such that tissue resistance also becomes least along the translatory planes (see Fig. 14). Finally, one determines tissue changes in response to deep inhalation or exhalation. It must be emphasized that excellent palpatory skills and great practice are indispensable for this technique.

After the point of greatest "ease," that is the point where the associated tissue resistance is least (tissue compliance the greatest), has been determined, the patient is held in that position for about 60-90 seconds. The muscles around the incriminated joint relax, allowing the joint to gain greater mobility. The new present neutral point is localized and the procedure is repeated again, up to a total of 3-4 times.

It is interesting and, yes, often surprising to the novice in this field of manual medicine to see how quickly a restriction responds to this form of treatment. Quite often it is perceived by the patient as one in which "not much happens." It has been our observation that especially patients who are used to associating an audible "cracking noise" with the success of treatment (i.e. during thrust procedures) are at first "disappointed" by the functional technique. After some time, however, and especially if subjective improvement is noted, the patient will be convinced of the procedure's effectiveness.

The functional technique is well suited for the anxious and nervous patient, as well as in acute situations for a patient with an overall poor health status. For instance, one may want to treat a myocardial infarction patient with this technique while he/she is still confined to the hospital, e.g. to treat a cervical lesion that causes the patient to have difficulty falling asleep and is thus keeping him from recovery.

4.3.2 Strain-Counterstrain Technique (After Jones)

The strain-counterstrain technique, like the functional technique, is a representative of the indirect treatment method. Furthermore, both of these techniques rely on a position of spontaneous release, which is in the direction toward immediate ease and comfort. In Jones' strain-counterstrain technique, however, and in contrast to the functional technique described above, a position of mild but asymptomatic strain is induced (rather than a bilateral balance of tension, Jones 1981). This concept embraces the principle that the most efficient reflex release will occur when the body or part is placed in a position of mild strain in a direction opposite to that in which the motion barrier is engaged (Ward 1981).

Jones identifies a set of what he calls tender points both anteriorly and posteriorly. He found that anterior tender points are present in dysfunctions eased by flexion, whereas posterior tender points are found in dysfunctions eased by extension. First, the individual tender point is identified by palpation. Then the point of greatest ease is introduced by placing that spinal area in a position of mild but asymptomatic strain (as described above). When the practitioner guides the incriminated joint and its associated muscles in the appropriate direction, again following along the planes of motion, the patient often reports immediately that he/she experiences decreased tenderness. At the point of greatest comfort the patient is held for 60-90 seconds, under constant monitoring of the accompanying tissue changes. The tender point ceases to cause discomfort to the patient the moment normal function is restored to the connective tissues associated with the incriminated joint.

In clinical practice, it is often necessary to resort to more than one technique when treating a patient. Depending on the individual clinical situation, the practitioner must be able to determine which is the most appropriate technique, and if necessary be able to alternate between the various techniques, as patient response is usually varied.

Both active and passive mobilization without impulse modalities can be used as an alternative to or as preparation for the mobilization techniques with impulse (low amplitude, high velocity thrust).

4.4 Low Amplitude, High Velocity Thrust Technique (Mobilization with Impulse)

It should be emphasized that specific manual therapeutic procedures such as the low amplitude, high velocity thrust technique should only be carried out by a qualified and trained practitioner who is licensed perform such procedures. The physician is able to make a diagnosis not only in regard to a specific manual medicine disorder, but he/she is able to evaluate the patient's overall health status at the time of the examination. Even though rare, complications can occur, and the physician must be able to immediately intervene so as to prevent a disastrous outcome. The different countries vary as to the personnel licensed to perform these specific procedures.

Thrust or mobilization with impulse techniques are viewed as perhaps the most elegant and quickest mode of releasing a restricted joint associated with a somatic dysfunction. Heilig (1981) describes the following three main features:

1) localization of the forces,
2) separation of joint surfaces, and
3) motion towards a barrier in the path indicated by the facet planes.

Execution of the procedure itself involves several steps:

1) correct patient positioning,
2) accurate localization of the joint at the barrier,
3) test pull (preparing the surrounding tissues),
4) complete patient relaxation,
5) impulse force (or low amplitude, high velocity thrust),
6) reevaluation.

It must be borne in mind that the preparation for the manipulative procedure requires more time and effort than the delivery of the impulse itself.

The patient is guided into as pain-free a position as possible. Naturally it is desirable that the practitioner him/herself is also relaxed so as to provide for calm and unharried movements.

According to Fryette's rule (page 32) the spinal segments above and below the incriminated segment are carried to their respective barriers, that is the "slack is taken out," and the joints are locked in that position. Thus, the restricted joint has been accurately localized and positioned so that the impulse force can act only on that one particular joint. The remaining spinal joints are therefore protected.

The practitioner's hands are placed close to the restricted joint, above the spinous and transverse processes of the specific spinal joint partner. The joint is carried carefully to the pathological barrier, in the path indicated by the three dimensional spatial arrangement of the joint's surface (flexion/extension, sidebending, rotation). Joint capsule and tendons at that joint are carefully stretched in the sense of "taking out the slack."

Between the engagement at the barrier and the delivery of the impulse force (thrust) one must wait a few seconds, that is remain in the "pre-tensing" period. Should the patient indicate aggravation of his/her symptoms or report any additional unpleasant sensation, such as vertigo, the therapeutic procedure must be terminated immediately and the patient reevaluated for the presence of any contraindication. Contraindications may include any inflammatory process, arthritis, vertebral artery compromise, etc. The period of preparation (pre-tension) can thus be viewed as a protective measure.

The patient's muscles should be completely relaxed during the time the impulse force is being delivered. Therefore, the patient is requested to deeply inhale and exhale. The operator follows the patient's respiratory cycle, and at the point of deepest exhalation delivers just enough of an impulse force to release the joint restriction.

The direction of impulse force is perpendicular or parallel to the tangential plane of the joint surface. The delivery of the force is of very short duration, about 10–100 msec (Young et al.). The capsule and tendons undergo mild stretch which is often accompanied by the well known "pop" or a "cracking" noise. Phonographically it is different from "normal cracking", e.g. that of a finger point (Lewit 1977). The amount of force that is delivered amounts to approximately 0.5-2% of the normal tensile strength of the healthy bone (Steglich 1974). The amount of force necessary is least when the joint has been accurately localized and the barrier correctly engaged. In some instances, appropriate positioning alone may bring about the resolution of a restriction.

The thrust technique can be handled in two ways depending on the pain behavior (see Fig. 56a, b). Treatment should always proceed in the *pain-free* direction. The quick stretch that is applied to the capsule and the tendons leads to a reflexive relaxation of the muscles associated with that joint (Hufschmidt in Terrier 1969; Eldred in Buerger 1979), which then allows improvement in joint congruity and ultimately in the resolution of the joint restriction. Thus the desired end result should be that of improvement in the patient's range of motion in the treated joint.

Should the patient indicate exacerbation of his/her pain while being guided towards the restrictive barrier, the procedure must follow the rules of the indirect techniques, that is treatment is in the opposite, the pain-free direction.

> Therapy always proceeds in the pain-free direction!

Somatic dysfunction never restricts movement along all planes simultaneously. One or several directions of movement remain free. If the patient, however, reports pain with positioning in all three planes, the thrust or impulse procedure must not be used at all, and the diagnosis should be reevaluated at that point. There may, for instance, be an inflammatory or destructive process which had not been previously identified.

The thrust or mobilization with impulse technique is applicable not only to the spinal joints but to the extremity joints as well. This technique, however, is rarely used for the larger joints, and if then mostly at the end of the mobilization treatment (i.e. attempting to treat the loss of about 5 degrees at the end range).

In contrast to the larger joints, the technique is applicable for restrictions involving the smaller extremity joints, such as the distal and proximal ulnar joint, the carpal-metacarpal and finger joints, tibia-fibular joint, and the joints of the ankle and foot.

Every treatment procedure must be followed by reevaluation. If the expected improvement or normalization of findings has not occurred with the treatment, one must guard against the temptation to repeat the same procedure, but applying a greater force. Be reminded that in clinical practice, too small a force has never been the cause of failure. It goes without saying that it is the duty of the treating physician to reevaluate the patient's previous diagnosis and the appropriateness of using this technique. In a certain number of cases one may come up with new indications for another technique, or contraindications to the thrusting technique. Thus the well trained physician is always prepared to formulate another treatment plan if indicated by the individual situation.

4.5 Other Techniques

Various other non-impulse techniques have been used in the field of manual medicine and include the myofascial release technique (Ward 1985) and the craniosacral technique.

4.5.1 Myofascial Technique

The myofascial release concept is a "combined approach" designed to assess and treat pathophysiological reflex mechanisms, soft tissue changes and faulty body mechanics anywhere in the body (Ward 1985). Therapeutic intervention is directed towards the restoration of myofascial continuity, integrity and symmetry. The approach, even though a more global one concentrating more often than not on entire body regions, can be utilized to treat specific segmentally occurring abnormalities.

4.5.2 Cranio-Sacral Technique

This technique, presented by W. H. Sutherland (Magoun 1976), refers to the management and therapy using manual medicine skills applied to the cranio-sacral rhythm (Briner 1981). This treatment technique, directed towards the cranium and sacrum, concentrates on possibly effecting shifts in circulation and pressure dynamics of the inherent motion of the cerebrospinal fluid. By applying pressure to the skull, the sacrum or both, pressure and frequency of the cycle are thought to be corrected. Refined palpatory skills and appropriate training are prerequisites for successful treatment. The technique can be applied in either a direct (against the resistant barrier) or an indirect (barrier disengagement) manner.

4.6 Reevaluation

The success of manipulative therapy depends not only on the appropriate treatment technique but also on the significance the somatic dysfunction plays in the overall disturbance of the musculoskeletal system and entire organism.

When the somatic dysfunction is the primary cause of the disturbance (i.e. acute torticollis) appropriate manual therapy will in most cases bring about an elegant and rather prompt therapeutic result. In certain cases the use of manual medicine techniques may need to be supplemented by physical medicine and/or pharmacologic intervention.

If the joint restriction is the result of other mechanical or reflexive changes in a joint, manual therapy may bring about some or even total, yet only temporary, relief to the patient by modifying the nociceptive afferent information. A lasting success will not be achieved, requiring that one treat the real cause of the problem, utilizing whichever therapeutic modalities that are called for by the individual joint problem.

If psychological factors play a role, such as stress at work, psychotherapy and counseling may become necessary, and one should always pay attention to the stressors in the patient's life.

> On the other hand, it is not rare for patients to be seen in our daily practice who have been subjected to batteries of countless treatment modalities, including pharmacological and physical therapy, only to realize that the expected outcome has not occurred. In many of these patients we have found a somatic dysfunction which responded to manual therapy with its soft tissue, mobilization and thrust techniques to be the underlying problem. The early diagnosis and correction of a disabling somatic dysfunction could save health insurance companies and the individual a significant amount of money and distress.

5 Contraindications to Manual Medicine

Somatic dysfunction with joint restriction, if clinically relevant, represents the indication for manual therapy. In the absence of a somatic dysfunction, manual therapy is not indicated. From this point of view, then, one is tempted to say that there exist no contraindications.

There are however, a number of clinical conditions which preclude the utilization of manual therapeutic intervention, and in particular the use of the high velocity, low amplitude thrust procedures (mobilization techniques with impulse). Contraindications to the non-impulse mobilization techniques appear to be very rare and have thus far not been reported in the literature (Greenman, Lewit, personal communications).

In any case, the *basic rule* of keeping the patient as *pain-free* as possible should always be adhered to when applying manual therapy.

Contraindications to manipulative procedures which have been reviewed in the literature include those enumerated by Kleynhans (1980), Grieve (1979) and Maitland (1977).

Included in the list of contraindications are vertebral malignancy, cauda equina syndrome, joint instability due to fractures and dislocations, severe degenerative joint disease and other rheumatological processes as well as spondyloarthropathies, hypermobility syndromes, osteomalacia and osteoporosis. The following entities will be described in more detail in the ensuing sections:

- inflammatory processes,
- destructive processes,
- trauma resulting in anatomical changes,
- severe forms of osteoporosis,
- degenerative changes,
- suspicion of or proven anomalies of the vertebral artery,
- certain psychological disturbances.

5.1 Inflammatory Processes

Manual therapy is not to be applied to joints that are acutely inflamed. After the inflammation has subsided, however, manual therapy can be utilized to resolve a possible remaining functional disturbance. This often brings about improvement in the range of motion in the particular joint, be it an apophyseal or extremity joint. The increase in range of motion thus achieved is often beneficial to the progress in physical therapy, as it may shorten the course of physical therapy. This may equally apply to cases where there is an especially long course of therapy, as for instance seen with Sudeck's atrophy or certain rheumatic diseases (i.e. ankylosing spondylitis).

At this point, it should be emphasized that manipulation and mobilization of the upper cervical joints in a patient with rheumatoid arthritis should be performed only in the rarest of instances and then with most extreme caution. Due to the possibility of weakening in the transverse ligament of the atlas and/or the alar ligaments there may be upper cervical spine instability. Manipulation in such a patient may have catastrophic results. The same caution is definitely indicated if the X-ray reveals the odontoid.

5.2 Destructive Processes

The mere suspicion of a tumor or metastatic spread is sufficient to preclude most of manual therapeutic procedures. If elicited through the history, further workup is necessary and should include the appropriate laboratory tests, radiographs, as well as CT scans and bone scans, MRI, etc., depending on the individual clinical situation.

5.3 Trauma with Associated Anatomical Changes

Manual therapy is not indicated in cases of joint subluxation and/or joint dislocation.

Less severe or minor trauma without anatomical injury is often accompanied by joint restriction due to the somatic dysfunction which may respond to manual therapy once the acute stage has subsided. For example, minor hand and wrist as well as foot and ankle sports injuries have shown good response to manual therapy.

"Whiplash" injury, a term more recently, and appropriately so, replaced by hyperextension/hyperflexion injury, is a special case. Even when the X-ray and functional radiological studies reveal no visible pathological change, one must in many cases assume that delicate bony fracture-resembling cracks, rupture of ligaments and/or other soft tissue injury has indeed occurred. It has proven useful to wait for a minimum of six weeks after the accident before manual therapy is started. It is important that the patient be reexamined at that time, and with contraindications excluded one may give careful manual treatment to any remaining somatic disturbances.

5.4 Osteoporosis

Depending on the severity of the disease, certain manual medicine techniques can be utilized. In the mild or less severe forms, a limited number of specific mobilization techniques have found application.

In severe forms, especially when there is vertebral wedging or "fish-mouth" vertebral changes, manual therapy is contraindicated. Painful positioning alone would in most cases prohibit even the gentlest of mobilization techniques.

5.5 Degenerative Changes

One of the frequently asked questions is whether manual therapy can be applied to joints that are affected by degenerative changes. Can it be applied to cases with disc problems? There have been cases in which the most significant degenerative changes affecting the apophyseal or extremity joints did not become symptomatic, with such a finding being rather a serendipitous one. It appears that the body is able to compensate for gradually progressing degenerative changes. A certain susceptibility, however, to dysfunction does exist.

Residual joint function may be preserved from the onset of degenerative changes up to shortly before there is complete joint stiffness. This residual function can in all stages be restricted by somatic dysfunction which, however, is amenable to manual therapy.

Naturally, the functional loss associated with the degenerative process remains unchanged.

Degenerative changes affecting a disc may not only alter the overall function in a spinal segment but may also contribute to and/or lead to somatic dysfunction. Manual therapy may alleviate some of the patient's pain if the secondary somatic dysfunction is treated successfully, despite the fact that the underlying cause has not been corrected. By correcting the function in a restricted apophyseal joint the body may be able to compensate for functional losses that are due to disc degeneration.

Disc herniation is an anatomical disruption with mechanical compression of a nerve root. Given the definition of somatic dysfunction or joint restriction, a herniated disc is *not* within the realm of manual therapeutic intervention. In many cases, however there exist simultaneous secondary somatic dysfunctions in the neighboring joints that are themselves amenable to manual therapy. In these situations mobilization and/or traction should be applied only.

It has been clinically noted that after disc surgery symptomatic joint dysfunction continues to be present in the lumbar spine and sacro-iliac joints. If manual therapy is indicated it may often relieve the patient from his/her "sciatica." Manipulation, however, should not be utilized until 6 weeks have elapsed after surgery.

5.6 Vertebral Artery

The vertebral artery has received special attention in the field of manual medicine. It has been known that thromboses that reach the vertebral artery can be caused by positioning of the patient's head in extension and some rotation (i.e. during intubation for anesthesia). Severe outcome and death after manipulation (thrust, impulse techniques) have been described in the literature (Schmitt 1978). Kleynhans (1980) in his extensive literature review of complications seen with manual therapy also reports cases where death has occurred due to vertebral artery injury. Dvořák and von Orelli (1982) report in a survey of 203 physicians in the Swiss Association for Manual Medicine: within the past 33 years approximately one and a half million manipulative procedures to the cervical spine have been performed. Complications were reported in 1248 cases, of which "vertigo" was reported in 1218 cases. In the remaining cases clouding or loss of consciousness and neurological deficits including tetraplegia occurred. According to the statistics presented in this study, there is a complication rate of 0.08% in manual treatments of the cervical spine, which is twice the rate reported in the American literature.

One must, however, suspect an even higher, albeit unknown, number of such complications that seem to occur exclusively with the thrust techniques (in contrast to the non-thrust mobilization techniques).

In daily practice, one of the most significant historical factors is "vertigo." One of the difficulties in obtaining a clear history is to exactly determine what the patient means by his "vertigo." It is the duty of the treating physician to exclude and, if indicated, work the patient up for causes related to the neurologic, vascular, ear, nose and throat or ophthalmological systems (Fig. 59).

Thrust or impulse techniques are absolutely contraindicated if the cause of the vertigo is a vascular one. Cervical vertigo, on the other hand, is one of the most rewarding indications of manual therapy, as the patient's symptoms frequently disappear, in many cases almost instantly. According to Tilscher (1977), 41% of vertigo has a cervical origin.

Various diagnostic procedures and tests can be utilized to differentiate among the various causes of vertigo (Hülse and Partsch 1976). Anomalies and changes affecting the vertebral arteries are more difficult to assess in an office setting. Various clinical tests have been proposed but are of rather limited value, including the hanging test by de Klejn (Fig. 60), and the Underberg-step test (Wolff 1983). Functional studies utilizing doppler sonography can at best indicate an artery lumen decrease greater than 50%. Arteriography as a screening test before manual therapy is not indicated and not without its own risks.

Hülse (1983) elaborated on the de Klejn's hanging test to differentiate between vascular and cervical vertigo. In this test, the cervical spine is slowly extended and then rotated to the left side followed by the right side. During this examination the patient wears a set of specific glasses with 20 diopters. If immediately on changing the positioning there is nystagmus which then goes on to resolve after a few seconds (decrescendo type), one is most likely dealing with a cervical vertigo. In such cases, manual therapy is indicated. If the nystagmus appears not until 20–30 seconds after positioning (crescendo type) and/or speech or consciousness changes become prominent, one is dealing with vascular vertigo. Returning the head and

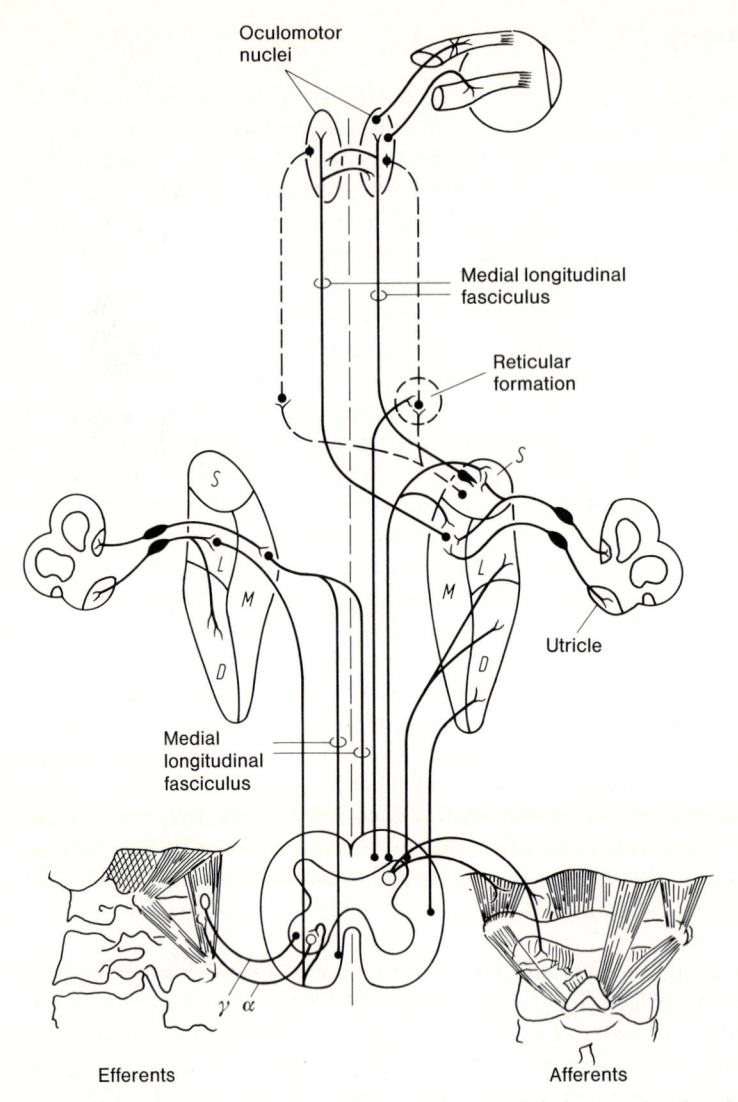

Fig. 59. Schematic representation of information transmission as related to the vestibular system. *S* superior vestibular nucleus; *M* medial vestibular nucleus; *D* inferior vestibular nucleus; *L* lateral vestibular nucleus. (After Wolff 1983)

cervical spine into the anatomical neutral position will generally alleviate the provoked signs. Manual therapy in this case is not indicated (Table 3).

How can complications involving the vertebral artery artery be prevented in manual medicine? In addition to a complete history and thorough examination it is recommended to only use active mobilization techniques. Thus far, complications of the vertebral artery secondary to the use of active mobilization techniques have not been described in the literature. These techniques, even though they are

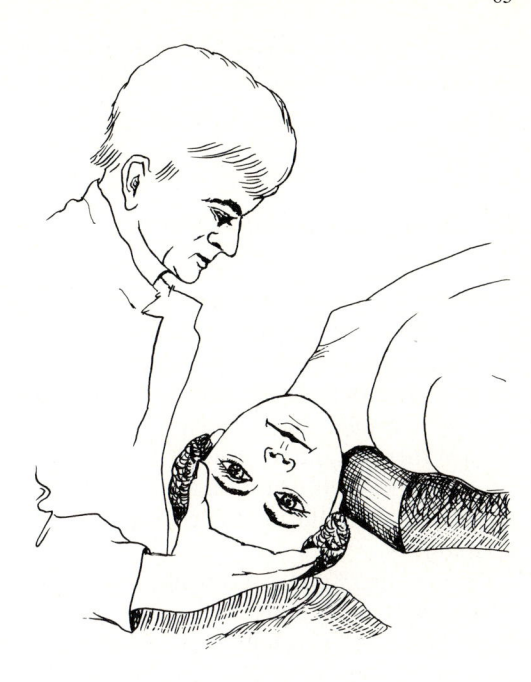

Fig. 60. The Kleijn hanging test which evaluates for compromise of the vertebral artery. (After Wolff 1983)

Table 3. Comparison between findings associated with vertebral-basal insufficiency and somatic dysfunction at the upper cervical spinal joints. (After Wolff 1983)

Vertebral-basilar insufficiency	Somatic dysfunction in upper cervical spinal joints
Episodes of syncope, "drop attacks," crescendo-type vertigo nystagmus *with* latency	Syncope is absent, no drop attacks decrescendo-type vertigo nystagmus *without* latency
de Klejn Hanging Test produces central symptoms towards end of movement, latency of 20-30 seconds, symptoms may become intolerable	*de Klejn Hanging Test* produces central symptoms the moment head and neck are moved, no latency, symptoms resolve with termination of test

being used more and more frequently by the physicians, can not always replace the thrust techniques.

Before applying manipulation to the cervical spine one should always introduce a "test traction." (p. 74) If the patient's symptoms are aggravated by the tractional force and/or if vertigo appears one should not utilize thrust techniques.

As described earlier manipulation should always be carried out in a routine, well organized, stepwise manner, starting with the correct and specific localization and positioning, followed by taking out the slack in the neighboring joints, introducing some preliminary tension (traction) force and then the well dosed (rather small) force or impulse. This technique should always be applied very carefully, especially when the treatment requires the cervical spine to be extended and simultaneously rotated. Overstretch and too great a force can be disastrous!

5.7 Psychological Disturbances

Psychological disturbances seem to play a significant role in causing neck and/or low back pain. Any type of exogenous or endogenous stress can be projected onto the spine, expressing itself as muscle tension changes and/or somatic dysfunction with joint restriction. One has to decide from case to case whether to use manual therapy to resolve the secondary joint dysfunction. It has been the experience that manual theray is often unsuccessful since the underlying disturbance continues to remain unresolved. Unfortunately there is always the danger and possibility that the physician could be made responsible for any exacerbation of the patient's symptoms.

On the other hand, successful treatment of the more chronic joint dysfunctions of the apophyseal joints in the spine may positively influence the patient and improve his overall psychological well being. Again it is clinical judgement that governs the decision whether treatment is indicated or not (see Fig. 1).

In practice, there is also a number of patients who become addicted to the "crack" often heard with the manipulative technique (which they interpret as the success of treatment). Furthermore, the relaxed state after treatment of a somatic dysfunction is found pleasant. Again, one must be very careful in treating such patients.

In summary, complications in manual medicine can be largely avoided by:

- well founded knowledge base and extensive training,
- thorough history and complete physical examination,
- correct indication,
- appropriate and case specific choice of treatment technique.

6 Hypermobility

6.1 General Hypermobility

We stated earlier that manual medicine concerns itself with the diagnosis and therapy of both segmental and peripheral articular dysfunction. A dysfunction is present not only when there is motion restriction, but can be caused by or associated with hypermobility as well. It is important to note that the treatment for the two situations is completely different.

Thus, in the broadest sense, manual therapy deals not only with the correction of motion restriction but also with the restoration of function in hypermobile, decompensated joints.

> Hypermobility in and of itself does not mean dysfunction.

There are people who, because of their innate constitution, possess an extremely flexible capsular and ligamentous apparatus with a greater than "normal" range of motion. We have all seen acrobats (i.e. the performing "rubber-" or "snake-man") who produce body contortions to an almost grotesque point. And it is not uncommon in certain highly competitive sports to make use of controlled hypermobility. Balanced and very specific training of certain muscles has been employed to improve overall performance; apparently this is felt to increase the action radius in such a manner that it improves technique, efficiency and flow of movement (Steinbrück and Rompe 1979).

Hormonal influences as they occur with pregnancy, for instance, may relax joint capsules, ligaments and tendons such that there is clinical hypermobility.

Sachse (1979) reviews the pathological forms of hypermobility associated with neuromuscular diseases.

General hypermobility is of specific importance to manual medicine since uncontrolled and/or abnormal hypermobility may lead to marked muscular imbalance and coordination problems which then can lead to secondary joint motion restrictions (somatic dysfunctions with decreased range of motion).

6.2 Local Pathological Hypermobility

In daily practice, it is not uncommon to encounter localized hypermobility, which must be appropriately diagnosed, since, as stated earlier, the treatment approach is entirely different from that for somatic dysfunctions associated with movement loss. However, it is important to remember that localized hypermobility can cause reflex changes somewhere else that are similar to those observed with somatic dysfunctions with motion restriction. Simply put, hypermobility in a spinal segment or peripheral joint is associated with greater than "normal" motion in one or more planes as well as an increase in joint play.

Causes for localized hypermobility include decompensated general hypermobility, abnormal or excessive loading forces on a joint, trauma and degenerative joint changes.

The diagnosis of hypermobility is made in the usual manner with a thorough history and general physical examination followed by specific localized (level) palpatory assessment (Stoddard 1970) being the key elements. The patient often complains about pain associated with assuming a certain posture for a longer period of time. The so called "cocktail-party syndrome" is but one example (Barbor 1979). Continuous car driving of long duration may also lead to pain which, however, should improve and may resolve when the patient moves.

Due to individual variation of joint mobility it is often difficult to determine whether a joint is abnormally hypermobile or still within the patient's normal range. In addition to the examination sequence described by Stoddard (1970) and a thorough examination of the neighboring joints, it is often necessary to very carefully palpate the ligamentous insertions at the hypermobile joints. These are points which are tender upon palpation and frequently are associated with swelling. In some clinical settings, it may become necessary to inject such tender points with a local anesthetic to see if the pain subsides. Diagnostically, it is also important to pay attention if the patient reports improvement after local anesthesia in any of the referred symptoms (i.e. pain in the posterior portion of the leg).

Jirout has successfully demonstrated hypermobility by using X-rays (quoted in Sachse 1979).

The treatment regimen for localized pathological hypermobility often may involve an entire set of treatment measures. Treatment-wise, it is easier to restore motion in a restricted joint than to bring a hypermobile joint into the state of adequate compensation. The primary goal is the prevention of further hypermobility. The patient who participates in any exercise regimen that results in or may contribute to progressive hypermobility must immediately stop such activities. Counseling about avoidance of abnormal posture and correct execution of activities of daily living (including at work) is one of the mainstays of appropriate treatment.

Mobilization which would lead to even greater mobility is naturally contraindicated. Nevertheless, as stated earlier, an originally hypermobile joint can also be restricted secondarily. In such cases treatment is very specific, gentle and well localized. It has been found clinically that an otherwise hypermobile joint which has lost some of its motion due to a restriction (secondary somatic dysfunction) can be successfully treated simply by engaging the joint's motion barrier.

Not rarely a decompensated hypermobile joint is found next to restricted joints. Careful and specific mobilization of the restricted joint may eliminate undue stress on the neighboring hypermobile joint. When balance or near balance of all the forces has been reached the patient may then report improvement or even relief of his/her symptoms.

In some cases it may become necessary to use immobilizing measures, such as bandages, splinting, pelvic belts or semielastic corsets. Isometric physical therapy (be reminded: no loosening exercises!) is the mainstay of therapy with the major goal being the improvement or resolution of muscular imbalance (Janda 1970). It is of utmost importance that the patient fully participates in his/her own treatment regimen on a daily basis.

Should all of these measures fail and the symptoms persist, one may want to resort to the fibro-osseous proliferation therapy described by Hackett (1956). It can be applied at any vertebral level but has found frequent utilization in the lumbosacral area. The sclerosing fluid (0.1 ml) is introduced at those areas of tenderness that coincide with the insertion of the tendon to the bone. The needle first makes contact with the bone at the insertion and is then somewhat withdrawn while fluid is being injected.

Hackett believed that through tissue proliferation one will induce a firming of the ligaments. Zicha (1979) seems to support this idea as demonstrated in his animal studies.

Lewit (1977) however believes that the effect actually results from a reduction of sensitivity at the tendon insertions secondary to the physical or chemical irritation and destruction of the nerve endings induced by the solution.

7 Cases from Clinical Practice

Joint dysfunctions can be the cause or result of an entire series of differing clinical presentations. Furthermore somatic dysfunctions may be incidental findings elicited in the physical examination. In addition to a thorough diagnostic workup the so called provisional treatment plan has proven very useful and effective. If, for example, a joint restriction is found in one or several apophyseal joints in a patient who presents with, for example, headache, back pain, or pain in the arm or chest wall, then the restriction should be treated. If this therapeutic intervention leads to a decrease or even the resolution of the patient's symptoms one may conclude that the joint dysfunction with its restriction was the cause or at least a significant contributor to the patient's symptoms. If the symptoms do not improve or recur soon after therapy other causes must be searched for.

This approach of using a provisional treatment plan is not only efficient but in many cases very cost effective. Unfortunately, and not too infrequently, patients come to our practice literally bringing with them stacks of medical records and X-ray films. And sadly enough, during the history it often becomes apparent that previously the patient's spine had not been palpatorily examined at all.

The following case descriptions represent only a selection of the more important and more frequently encountered clinical presentations amenable to manual therapy.

7.1 Cervical Syndrome

The term "cervical syndrome," a term used mostly in Europe, is nothing but a catch-all description revealing only that the cervical spine is involved. It says nothing about the type and nature of symptoms. In clinical practice, however, it has become customary to subdivide the cervical syndrome further into the so called "upper syndrome" (C0–C3) and the "lower syndrome" (C4–C7).

7.1.1 Upper Cervical Syndrome

The patient complains of headache, dizziness, visual and auditory changes, occasionally about the feeling of swelling in the throat (Seifert 1981). Various causes can be listed for these symptoms. According to our experience, in more than 50% of the cases we see with such presenting complaints the cause can be attributed to a joint dysfunction in the cervical spine, be it the primary or secondary cause. According to Tilscher (1977), dysfunctions associated with joint restriction in the upper cervical spine account for 50% of the occurrence of headaches and 40% of dizziness.

If the patient presents with shoulder, neck or arm pain it has become routine to seek for causes in the cervical spine. This is not the case when the patient presents with headache, dizziness, chest pain or fullness in the throat. It is therefore not surprising to see that a patient with such symptoms has undergone a whole series of different examination procedures and treatments. It is often not until the patient has had full neurologic, internal medicine, ENT or ophthalmological evaluation and therapeutic trials that the cervical spine is considered as the responsible factor. In many cases a manual examination with simple palpation and without complex equipment will then a somatic joint dysfunction in the upper cervical spine to be responsible for the patient's presenting complaints.

One of the major tasks is to determine whether the dysfunction is the primary cause of the upper cervical syndrome or if it is the secondary result of a disturbance in the patient's anatomy or reflexive neuro-regulatory processes associated with the spinal segments. In other words, we must determine whether the dysfunction is the "conductor" or a "player" in the pathological "orchestra." The success of therapy is governed by this decision.

Manual therapy as it applies to this particular spinal area may be illustrated by the following practical examples.

Somatic Dysfunction with Joint Restriction as the Primary Cause

Movement Imbalance
The patient was a 38-year-old male with a lower extremity prosthesis and poor gait pattern. The patient reported that upon rising from an armchair he perceived "a jerk" in his neck. This was accompanied by a sudden onset of dizziness with every movement of the head. The patient was evaluated by seven different specialists before being referred by an internist for manual medicine evaluation of the spine.

Examination revealed an atlas restriction. The patient became symptom-free after one manipulative treatment.

"Malpositioning"
A 65-year-old female was seen in the office because of a levator-scapulae-tendinopathy. Incidentally she remarked that on the same day she was to be admitted in the hospital's ENT service because of sudden loss of hearing. She stated she had "slept wrong" the previous night.

Manual examination revealed an atlas restriction which responded immediately to manipulative therapy. During the subsequent admission examination in the hospital, no sign of the previous hearing disturbance could be found.

Joint Restriction Secondary to a Mechanical Disturbance

Faulty Posture at the Job Site
A 65-year-old dentist complained of double vision which had suddenly developed approximately four weeks prior to his visit. Examinations by an ophthalmologist, neu-

rologist and ENT specialist were noncontributory. The patient also underwent acupuncture as well as injection therapy, both of which were unsuccessful. He then remembered that concurrent with the double vision he had been experiencing neck pain. These emerged after having purchased a new treatment chair which required him to alter his working posture.

Manual medicine examination revealed joint restriction at C1-C2. Two days after one manipulation treatment the double vision had resolved. The dentist returned to using his previous treatment chair, eliminating the mechanical cause of his somatic dysfunction. There was no recurrence of the problem.

Abnormal Loading Forces
A 46-year-old car salesman complained about a 15 year history of intermittent, periodic episodes of acute cephalgia. He had not been able to identify any precipitating factors. The patient stated that the headaches had previously been treated as migraine headaches.

Manual medicine examination revealed a somatic dysfunction at C1-C2 on the left and an asymmetric pelvis. Lumbar, pelvic and hip X-rays utilizing the Gutmann technique (p. 56) showed the sacral base to be tilted inferiorly by 1 cm on the left. The restrictions at the neck and pelvis were treated using manual medicine techniques, and the patient was instructed to wear a heel lift. He became symptom free after two treatment sessions. At a later time he forgot to place the required heel lift in his newly purchased pair of shoes and the headaches recurred. These disappeared with placement of the heel lift in the new shoes.

Somatic Dysfunction Secondary to Psychological Disturbances

Psychosomatic
A 35-year-old female came to the office because of a long-standing history of shoulder and neck pain which also radiated to the head. Examination revealed significant muscle tension in the neck and shoulder muscles along with a segmental restriction at C0-C1 and C5-C6. The patient underwent manual therapy with subsequent physical therapy and antiinflammatory medication. The joint restrictions, however, recurred frequently after short intervals of temporary improvement. Again a detailed history was obtained which now revealed significant marital discord and financial difficulties. Further manual therapy was not undertaken and the patient was referred for psychological assessment and therapy.

Space Occupying Lesion
Quite impressive is the case of a 48-year-old male salesman who was referred to this office by his internist because of a one week history of headaches. A thorough examination by the internist had not revealed the cause of the headaches, and a cervical syndrome was suspected. Manual examination revealed a C1-C2 joint restriction which originally responded well to manual therapy. Two weeks later the patient developed the same symptoms with the same diagnostic findings. Again therapy was successful, albeit only for a short period of time, as soon thereafter the patient again developed repeated headaches. Reexamination at that time did not reveal joint restriction. The patient was then referred to a neurologist who found no indications of a brain tumor. One week later the patient required hospitalization after his internist

diagnosed papilledema. Subsequent craniotomy revealed metastatic bronchial carcinoma in the posterior cranial fossa. Subsequent chest radiographs did not disclose the primary tumor.

This case shows that manual therapy may be able to resolve secondary joint dysfunctions thus making it easy to overlook and search for the existence of a primary cause. This is a trap one must always be aware and wary of!

7.1.2 Lower Cervical Syndrome

The lower cervical syndrome is also known as the cervicobrachial syndrome as the pain frequently radiates into the arms as well.

The patient usually complains of pain originating in the neck and radiating, mostly unilaterally but also bilaterally, into the shoulder, elbow and occasionally into the hand. In some cases the patient complains of isolated shoulder, elbow or hand pain which may be solely due to vertebral dysfunction which should always be included in the differential diagnosis. First of all, however, one must exclude any radicular etiology. Segmental joint restriction and irritation is easy to palpate. Peripheral segmental irritation can be found in the hyperalgetic zones as they relate to the associated dermatomes, but in much less distinct and clear delineation than is the case with nerve root compression. For further orientation one can utilize the so called "identification muscles" as described by Hansen and Schliack (1962). These muscles when palpated can have higher tone, or present as a palpable band and as myotendinosis.

Specifically, the following distinction is made:
- C4–C5: Pain is localized anteriorly from the shoulder to the elbow crease.
    Muscles affected: deltoid, supraspinatus, infraspinatus and teres minor muscles.
    Possible concomitant involvement: there may be periarthritis of the shoulder.
- C5–C6: Pain is localized anteriorly at the shoulder, lateral side of the arm and thumb.
    Muscles affected: biceps and brachioradialis muscles.
    Possible other involvement: lateral epicondylitis, styloiditis of the radius.
- C6–C7: Pain is localized posteriorly at the shoulder, the arm, index, middle and ring fingers.
    Muscles affected: triceps brachii.
    Possible other involvement: medial epicondylitis.
    Differential diagnosis: carpal tunnel syndrome.
- C7–C8: Pain is localized to the medial side of the arm, ring finger and little finger.
    Muscles affected: hypothenar muscles.
    Differential diagnosis: ulnar carpal tunnel syndrome.

Again, there is a good amount of segmental variation. Individual segmental variation of about one segmental level has been described in 20% of the population.

Because neck and/or arm pain are one of the frequent presenting complaints it is important to have a good understanding of the relationship between neck and arm pain.

Vice versa, there may be cases in which disturbances originating in the arm and shoulder are projected towards the spine. Brügger (1977) reports a case in which a chronic cervical syndrome resolved after surgical removal of a ganglion in the wrist. For example, it would not be inappropriate to examine the spine when the presenting complaint is apparently the result of an epicondylitis. This is of importance especially when the concomitant or causative somatic joint dysfunction is clinically silent. It is necessary to address any and all sources of dysfunction, so as to guarantee continued normal functioning of the musculoskeletal system.

7.2 Thoracic Syndrome

From a manual diagnostic and therapeutic standpoint the thoracic spine has a number of special features that need to be mentioned.

In contrast to the other spinal areas, where one spinal segment is made up of two joint partners, there are two paired joint partners that relate to one thoracic spinal segment, consisting of the paired apophyseal joints and rib joints. The components of the rib joint, the costotransverse and costovertebral joint, form a functional unit which is clinically assessed as such. Whereas the apophyseal joints are innervated by the dorsal ramus of the spinal nerve, the rib joints are innervated by the ventral ramus of the spinal nerve (Wyke 1979).

It is important to separate out joint dysfunctions related to the apophyseal joint from dysfunctions associated with the rib joint as the treatment techniques are not the same for both. This is especially important as the symptoms may be much the same.

Joint dysfunction at the apophyseal or rib joints are common causes for arm pain, pain in the back and between ribs, as well as general upper thoracic discomfort.

An example:

A 37-year-old secretary with a tendency towards hypermobility reported a history of years of complaints in the neck and thoracic region, especially after overexertion at her job or when participating in sports (tennis). Manual therapy and irregular physical therapeutic exercises had provided some symptomatic relief for longer periods of time. The patient suffered another acute, this time quite severe, attack which resulted in her being admitted to the neurological unit in the hospital because her family physician suspected either a space occupying lesion or inflammatory/destructive process. The usual workup, including myelography, could not determine the cause for the patient's symptoms. A diagnosis of neuralgia was made, and after a extensive trial of various medications had failed, the permanent use of TENS units was recommended, with the intention to somehow block the pain electrically. During visiting hours, her husband elected to take her to a physician trained in manual medicine for further consultation (without informing the physician of the fact that the patient was still officially an inpatient).

In the examination at the office a group lesion at T1-T2-T3 on the right side with flexion, rotation and left sidebending restriction was diagnosed. Furthermore the patient's right first rib resisted exhalation, while the second and third ribs on the right had an inhalation restriction. Utilizing various soft tissue techniques and active mobilization maneuvers, in particular the muscle energy technique, the patient reported significant relief. Two days later she was discharged from the hospital pain-free.

Of particular interest is the close relationship between the somatic and *autonomic* nervous system in the thoracic spine. Dysfunctions can arise either from the spine and thoracic wall directly or be influenced by the internal organs such as the heart, vessels and lung as well as others in the thoracic cavity (Stiles 1979; Kunert 1975; Bergsmann and Eder 1967; Wyke 1979; Beal 1983).

In clinical practice a connection between cardiac symptoms and dysfunctions of the apophyseal joints between C5 and T4 and the related rib joints has been observed. The symptom common to the various disorders is chest wall pain which may be due to one of the following (as well as a combination thereof):

1) Segmental restriction between C5 and T4 and/or the associated rib joints. The pain is projected to the precordial area of the thorax. Organic cardiac disease has been ruled out. Manual medicine removes the primary disturbance, which is musculoskeletal in this case.
2) Concomitant joint restriction between C5 and T4 may occur in the presence of e.g. ischemic heart disease. This is true for the corresponding rib joints and the shoulder joints as well. These restrictions are therefore secondary to an organic disease. They are mediated via neurogenic reflex patterns and occasionally may persist beyond the time when therapy for the cardiac disease has been completed. Manual therapy is then indicated. If the patient's secondary restrictions are not recognized as such and if symptoms continue to exist, there is great danger that the patient's complaints will be classified as "non-real," or as psychogenic.
3) The summation of various simultaneous stimuli from different sources, each of which would be below its modality specific threshold, can lead to clinical symptoms (Korr 1975). With a certain predisposition to cardiac disease, arrhythmias may be associated with somatic dysfunctions arising from the C5 to T4 spinal segments. Such dysrhythmias usually resolve after appropriate manual therapy. The individual stimulation from one source would have been below the threshold to cause a nocireaction.

Schwarz (1970) reports a case where dysrhythmias became apparent whenever there was a simultaneous joint dysfunction at the cervico-thoracic junction. In studies using ECG recordings, he demonstrated the disappearance of the dysrhythmia to be concurrent with the resolution of the somatic dysfunction.

The above examples of "cardiac symptoms" can be applied to other organs and organ systems as well, including abdominal and genitourinary disturbances. Thus knowledge of these correlations *are* of great practical clinical significance but unfortunately have received too little attention.

These findings may be of particular interest to the internist and cardiologist, who, once diseases of cardiac origin have been ruled out, may want to examine the spine routinely for paravertebral tender points, limiting time consuming and expensive examination procedures to a minimum.

7.3 Lumbar Syndrome

A great number of causes have been incriminated as responsible for the chronic lumbar syndrome. Two causes frequently observed in the daily practice of a practitioner of manual medicine are *abnormal loading forces* and *muscular imbalance*.

The degree of inappropriate loading forces and thus static aberrations when the patient is standing is best evaluated utilizing the lumbar-pelivs-hip X-ray studies recommended by Gutmann (1975a, p. 56).

The lateral view allows evaluation of the longitudinal axis of the sacrum in the sagittal plane. One distinguishes between two arrangements, the so called "flat back" type and the "arched back" type.

In the flat back type, the sacrum's longitudinal axis is rather vertical (the sacral base is correspondingly more horizontal). In contrast, in the arched back type, the sacrum's longitudinal axis is more towards the horizontal (albeit, the sacral base is more vertical, pointing anteriorly). The steep angle type (=flat back) is associated more frequently with hypermobility, whereas the shallow angle type tends to be associated with motion restriction. The arched back type has also been known as the "overstrain" type (Fig. 61 a, b).

In the antero-posterior projection one is able to evaluate the level of femoral heads, sacral base, pelvic crest level and any lateral spinal deviations (Fig. 62).

The antero-posterior views are very helpful in evaluating the standing patient and any structural changes resulting from faulty static loading forces. Heufelder (1983) reports that 63.37% of 700 patients whose chief complaint was back pain had a leg length difference, asymmetry of the ilium or dysplasia at the lumbar-sacral spine level. Friberg (1983) examined 266 recruits in Finland. In more than 50% of the subjects he found a leg length difference of greater than 5 mm evident on X-ray. 18% of the recruits had a leg length difference greater than 10 mm and 3% had a difference exceeding 15 mm. Compared to a symptom-free control

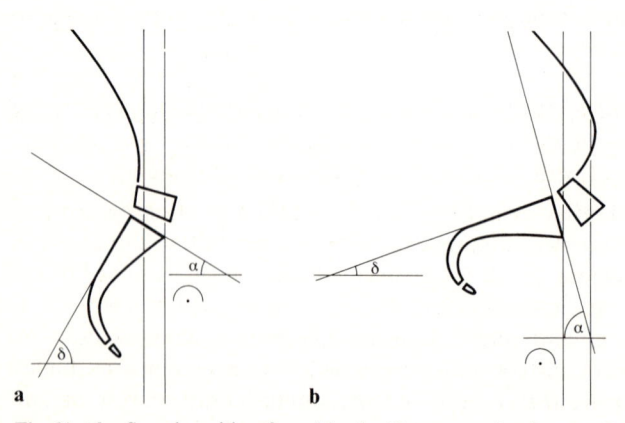

Fig. 61 a, b. Sacral position found in the X-ray examination: **a** flat back **b** arched back

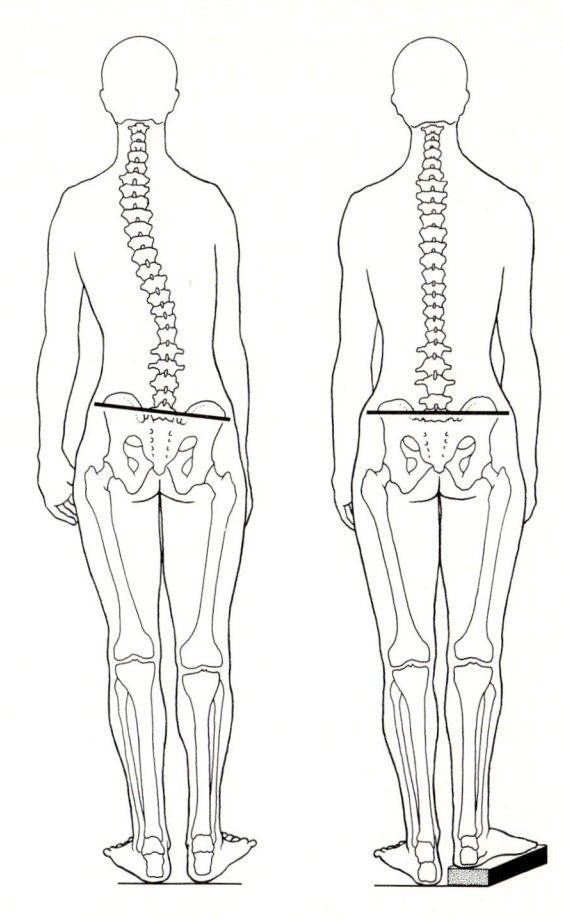

Fig. 62. Postural correction in the frontal plane by leveling the sacral base. (After Lanz-Wachsmuth 1982)

group, the frequency of leg length difference was 2 to 5 times greater in a group of patients with complaints of chronic back pain ranging from 14–89 years.

This is in agreement with the observation made by practitioners of manual medicine who found that asymmetries discernible on frontal X-rays – which are associated with faulty loading forces – may significantly contribute to chronic low back pain. In many cases a prescription for the lift of a heel is indicated. According to Niethard (1982) a small lift may even be necessary in clinical cases with less substantial loading abnormalities. More important than level and symmetry of the femoral head and the pelvic crest is the sacral base on which the lumbar spine rests (Greenman 1979a). The sacral base should be parallel to the lower edge of the X-ray film, again utilizing exactly the criteria proposed by Gutman (p. 56). Greenman (1979a) draws a line tangential to the sacral base from edge to edge and then constructs a line perpendicular to it through either apex of the femoral head. The measured difference is equal to the height of heel lift required for the patient. Other measurements utilizing tape measure, water-level gauge, as well as trial and error associated with placement of various height heel lifts all seem too imprecise as they do not take into account the level of the sacral base. This may be one of the reasons why there exist such diverse opinions about the need for heel lifts.

The sacral base plane can be unleveled not only by anatomical disorders but also for functional reasons, e.g. somatic dysfunction of a sacro-iliac or a lumbar apophyseal joint. All functional lesions must be treated first, before the lifting of a heel is taken in consideration.

If the sacral base in a patient with recurrent symptoms is anatomically unlevel the placement of a heel lift is indicated when the side to side difference is 0.5 cm or greater. However, with asymmetries greater than 0.5 cm heel lift prescription proceeds gradually. According to Rompe (1978) the heel lift should not be increased by more than 0.5 cm every six months. The goal of heel lift placement is as good and full a compensation as possible. In an elderly patient with compensatory scoliosis, for instance, or in the presence of degenerative changes, partial compensation is the goal.

In some cases, Greenman (1979a) has found it necessary to place a heel under the longer leg as well so as to bring about a leveling of the sacral base.

Another common cause of chronic low back pain and recurrent somatic dysfunctions associated with the apophyseal joints is *muscular imbalance* in the lumbar, pelvic and hip region (p. 59). The muscles should routinely be examined for weakening and shortening. Manual muscle testing not only for strength but also for changes in length is indispensable in the diagnostic workup and the evaluation of the treatment success.

The best preventative measures against chronic low back pain and other functionally related spinal disturbances are:

1) continued use of a heel lift if indicated, in any shoe the patient wears (dress shoes, sneakers, etc.),
2) daily exercise program specific for the individual patient and his/her muscular imbalance problems,
3) physiologically correct posture in activities of daily living and at work (Eklundh 1979; Stoddard 1982).

7.4 Sciatica

7.4.1 Differential Diagnosis of Lumbar Disc Herniation

Not all pain radiating into the leg is due to prolapse of a lumbar intervertebral disc. In the daily practice of the physician who engages in manual medicine leg pain is due to the following causes, listed in descending order of frequency of occurrence:

> Sacro-iliac joint restriction, apophyseal joint restriction in the lower lumbar spine, ligamentous insufficiency, lumbar disc protrusions and/or prolapse, coccydynia, inflammatory or destructive processes.

Apart from inflammatory or destructive processes which should be excluded during the course of the patient's general health evaluation, it is important to differentiate whether the low back pain and the associated leg pain is most likely due to a prolapsed disc or a segmental somatic dysfunction. Once the decision has been made as to the possible etiology, treatment can proceed which is naturally very different for the different causes. In the case of a suspected disc prolapse, manual therapy is not indicated, whereas if the cause is felt to be due to a somatic dysfunction manual therapeutic intervention is the treatment of choice. In some cases, however, manual therapy can come into play when there is a somatic dysfunction coexistent with a disc problem.

Steinrücken (1980) devised a table to aid in the differential diagnosis of prolapsed disc. Table 4 presented here is a modified version. This table may help the physician not trained in manual medicine to identify possible somatic dysfunctions. This may expedite the referral to a manual medicine practitioner who then utilizes specific and rather refined examination techniques so as to come to a precise diagnosis and initiate the appropriate therapeutic intervention plan. Thus, in appropriate cases expensive CT (computer tomograph) or even MRI (magnetic resonance imaging) may be avoided.

Differential diagnosis may be complicated in a good number of cases of low back and leg pain, as radicular symptoms may not be present alone but rather coexist and thus blur with simultaneous pseudoradicular symptoms due to reflexively mediated somatic dysfunctions arising from the lower lumbar spine or the sacro-iliac joints. In such cases it is not only very important to closely observe patient response to therapy but additional diagnostic investigations using such modalities as myelography, CT scanning or MRI may be in order.

7.4.2 Sacro-iliac Joints

In daily practice, sacro-iliac joint dysfunction is a frequent cause of both acute and chronic low back complaints. The patient often complains about pain which radiates to the posterior thigh.

Up until a few years ago little was known and little attention was paid to sacro-iliac dysfunctions in the traditional fields of medicine. Physicians were primarily trained to pay attention only to diagnosis and treatment of trauma and destructive and inflammatory processes involving this joint. The patient's symptoms were diagnosed generally as "sciatica." Later, a better understanding of sacro-iliac joint motion both during standing and in movement was gained by applying very refined and specific manual medicine examination procedures. One was therefore able to use distinctive criteria that would aid in the examination of a patient with

Table 4. Differential diagnosis of ruptured lumbar disc (RLD)

Signs/symptoms indicating RLD	Signs/symptoms indicating other possible causes, i.e. somatic dysfunction
Pain radiates in segmental (dermatomal) distribution	Pain radiation is more or less diffuse
Pain is exacerbated by Valsalva maneuver, coughing, sneezing	Pain is rarely exacerbated by Valsalva maneuvers. Increased vibration associated with coughing or sneezing may cause localized pain exacerbation
Certain movements cause "electric shock"-like discomfort	Specific movements may in some cases cause radiating pain into the leg, but more often are associated with localized exacerbation; electric shock-like pain is rare
Pain may have neuralgia-like character, worse with sitting	Pain may improve with sitting
Objective findings, patient standing: Protective posture, secondary scoliosis, frequently towards the non-involved side. Compensation to correct for abnormal loading conditions has not occurred. Head plumb-line shifted from foot plumb-line	Protective posture often present, but correction/compensation for abnormal loading conditions has taken place
Sidebending towards the involved side and extension in spine cannot be performed due to pain inhibition; attempt of these movements causes pain to radiate into the leg	Sidebending towards involved side cannot be performed, or if it can, then only in limited manner due to pain inhibition. Pain may on occasion radiate into the leg. Pain is often localized
Objective findings, patient supine: Lasègue test positive at <45 degrees; sharp shooting pain elicited with test	Lasègue test positive at >50 degrees; pain increases gradually, so called "Pseudo-Lasègue"
Crossed Lasègue test positive	Crossed Lasègue test negative, even when there was unilateral limitation due to pain inhibition
Manual muscle testing may reveal weakness in segmentally related muscles	Muscle weakness is reported by patient but not objectively demonstrated
Reflexes decreased or absent	Reflexes usually present
Decreased or absent sensory perception to pain or light touch in dermatomal distribution	Increased sensory perception to pain in some dermatomes; Kibler skin rolling may be painful
Objective findings, patient prone: Pain perception upon pressure of incriminated spinous process	Pain perception upon pressure onto lateral portion of the spinous process
"Door bell" phenomenon: palpatory pressure upon the paraspinal muscles induces sharp pain shooting into the leg	Predominantly localized pain with palpation; springing test is usually negative
Pain perception to palpation at typical "sciatic points" (according to Valleix)	Tender points may be associated with changes in muscle texture (increased tension) or changes at the tendon's insertion of the muscle associated with the incriminated joint(s)

complaints of low back and leg pain. Once established as a sacro-iliac joint dysfunction specific therapeutic maneuvers could be applied.

Similar to the other components of the musculoskeletal system described thus far, dysfunctions arising from the pelvic girdle and the sacro-iliac joint in particular can be grossly categorized as either motion restriction or pathological hypermobility (p. 85).

As we have mentioned on p. 25, there is no active movement at the sacro-iliac joint. When bending forward, that is introducing flexion to the lumbar spine, the sacrum undergoes concomitant anterior movement (as it is suspended between the ilia), which in the literature has been termed "nutation" movement. During the walking cycle the sacrum alternately rotates about one or the other diagonal axis (Fig. 14), depending on the phase of walking (stance versus swing leg). Any of the different sacro-iliac joint movements can be restricted clinically.

Trauma can cause additional motion abnormalities different from those just described. The following abnormalities exist:

1) The so called *"upslip"* in which the entire half of the pelvis has moved superiorly; example: missing a step when descending.
2) The so called *"downslip"*, in which the entire half of the pelvis has moved inferiorly; examples: fall during skiing after the binding has not released; falling off a horse with one leg caught in the stirrup; there have been reports that even forceps delivery may cause a downslip in the mother.
3) The so called *"outflare"* in which the entire half of the pelvis has been moved laterally.
4) The so called *"inflare"* in which the entire half of the pelvis has been moved medially; example: after a fall landing on the involved hemipelvis; vaginal delivery may cause such a dysfunction.

Again, as stated earlier, it is simply not good enough to diagnose the existence of a dysfunction. One must be able to diagnose the type and direction of a somatic joint dysfunction. The following example may serve as an illustration:

A 42-year-old, slender, graceful, female gymnastics instructor with a tendency towards hypermobility landed on the "wrong foot" when dismounting from the gymnastics apparatus. During the subsequent days she developed back pain which was radiating increasingly into the left leg. Neurologic examination was unremarkable. Conservative treatment including massage, hot packs, electrotherapy, traction, local infiltration and antiinflammatory medications was without the desired result. The patient then underwent myelography on two different occasions (!) which did not demonstrate any compression or other changes. It was then recommended to the patient to undergo exploratory surgery with the intention of opening the lumbar spinal canal. The patient then visited a physician trained in manual medicine. Examination again did not reveal any neurologic deficits. Specific manual muscle testing, evaluating both length and strength, revealed shortening of the left hamstrings (termed "pseudo-Lasègue"), a positive flexion test on the left and sacro-iliac upslip. Manual treatment was followed by almost complete relief. Two days later, however, the patient experienced a recurrence when during a gymnastics exercise she tried, while supine, to reach with her legs for a ball over her head. This time the sacrum was diagnosed to have rotated anteriorly and inferiorly in the form of a left torsion. Manual treatment was successful in resolving the restriction and a pelvic belt was prescribed to prevent the patient from further relapse. She subsequently remained asymptomatic.

The field of manual medicine can be given credit for identifying functional abnormalities in the sacro-iliac joint, facilitating the understanding of the complex nature of the lower lumbar syndrome, and providing specific diagnostic and therapeutic guidelines.

7.4.3 Coccydynia

A functional disturbance arising from a dysfunction of the coccyx is a frequently overlooked cause of low back pain. This dysfunction is often associated with pain radiating to either or both thighs and has been extensively described by Lewit (1977) and colleagues from the Prague school (Manca et al. 1977). The patient's complaints center around pain especially when sitting on a hard surface. There may or may not be a history of a fall or difficult vaginal delivery. Specific palapatory examination and in certain cases the addition of a digital rectal examination will reveal the source of pain. In some cases the muscles at the coccyx are so tense that mobilization and/or manipulation is not sufficient and must be supplemented by infiltration therapy either directly at the tender point or through the sacral canal.

7.5 Extremity Joints

Manual medicine has significantly contributed to and expanded our understanding of extremity joint function, refining the diagnostic process and providing specific treatment techniques. It has become routine to not only examine the particular capsular pattern of a joint at hand but also evaluate coordination abnormalities of the muscles as they relate to that joint. Furthermore, the evaluation of joint play takes on a significant role in the diagnosis, as the subtle findings elicited aid more in the diagnosis than any other examination technique. The example presented here may serve as illustration:

A 45-year-old nurse reported a 6 month history of pain at the left foot with no apparent trauma. She was seen by an orthopedist who diagnosed a flat foot syndrome.

After a cast mold she received arch supports made of leather and cork, however without appreciable relief. Radiological studies were unremarkable. She then received repeated steroid injections into the most tender point at the instep, again providing temporary relief only. The orthopedist then consulted a physician trained in the manual examination and treatment of extremity joints.

Repeat examination revealed a "normal" flat foot. Standard motion testing demonstrated normal joint mobility in all joints including the ankle joint and the metatarsophalangeal joints. There was significant point tenderness over the navicular bone.

Specific manual medicine examination, however, revealed a restriction of gliding movement and diminished joint play between the navicular bone and the cuneiform bone of the great toe. After a number of passive mobilizations the joint was manipulated with a low amplitude, high velocity thrust procedure. This was associated with a loud cracking sound. Repeat motion testing revealed normal joint movement. The patient became symptom-free after two days once the period of irritation had subsided.

Many causes can be cited for functional abnormalities at the extremity joints. These may include chronic abnormal posture, prolonged immobilization such as occurs with a cast, minor trauma (abnormal reaching for an object, sprain/strains, etc), overuse through sports, joint disease such as rheumatoid arthritis or Sudeck's atrophy, joint degeneration etc.

Manual therapy to the extremity joint is actually very gentle, as the direction of treatment is either perpendicular or tangential to the joint's surface, avoiding strain to the ligaments and joint capsules.

Diminished joint play due to a somatic joint restriction may be treated by either mobilization techniques or manipulative (thrust) techniques. Angular movement is normalized by freeing up the translatory movement. Again and again the practitioner will be surprised by the scope and treatment successes achieved with the manual medicine modalities. Furthermore, the techniques as they apply to the extremity joints elegantly provide immediate relief in even some of the more stubborn cases.

Again, another example may illustrate this point:

A 50-year-old electrician fell onto his right shoulder in a skiing accident with subsequent development of a frozen shoulder. Conservative treatment was initiated. Hot packs exacerbated the patient's symptoms. Massage, diathermy, intraarticular cortisone injections, oral antiinflammatory agents, sedatives and stellate ganglion blocks did not bring about any relief. Physiotherapy was terminated because of severe pain.

Five months after the accident the patient was seen as an outpatient in one of the ambulatory care clinics at a university hospital. The physician who saw the patient had just finished one of the manual medicine courses about extremity joints. He found the right shoulder to be totally stiff. Only 20° of internal rotation had remained intact. After treatment utilizing traction the patient reported some relief as well as some improvement in mobility. Internal rotation had improved by 10°. Now there was also 10° of abduction. The previously scheduled manipulation procedure under anesthesia was deferred and a conservative treatment plan was initiated. For a period of nine weeks the patient received daily traction and translatory mobilizations. The shoulder gained full range of motion by the end of this treatment regimen.

Manual therapy to the extremity joints is not a monotherapy. It is indicated when, due to a functionally reversible abnormality, that is a somatic joint dysfunction, there is change from the normal capsular pattern and abnormal joint play in the incriminated joint. Treatment of extremity joint dysfunction is supplemented by the appropriate use of nonsteroidal antiinflammatory agents, as well as physical medicine and therapeutic rehabilitation interventions. Manual therapy not only facilitates the work of the therapist but also speeds up the patient's return to as normal a level of functioning as the individual case allows.

8 Afterword

This book is intended to provide the reader with a general overview of the current scope and status of manual medicine. The author hopes that each reader will be stimulated to learn more about this exciting field, and if not at least to have been provided with a basis for critical discussion and an educated opinion.

Those wishing to obtain a better understanding of the field of manual medicine are encouraged to familiarize themselves with the subject matter through the standard texts and better yet by enrolling in the various practical courses offered by the different institutions.

Manual medicine is a practical, "hands on" specialty field in medicine. Even if one were able to produce the clearest and most useful descriptions and diagrams, they could never come close to replacing the experience and skills gained from actually touching the patient. As in many other fields of knowledge, practice makes perfect.

9 References

Andersen B (1982) Stretching. Shelter Publications. Bolinas, California
Arlen A (1979) Biometrische Röntgenfunktionsdiagnostik an der Halswirbelsäule. Fischer, Heidelberg (Schriftenreihe Manuelle Medizin, vol 5)
Barbor R (1979) Instabilität der Wirbelsäule. Theoretische Fortschritte und praktische Erfahrungen der Manuellen Medizin. Konkordia, Bühl, pp 172–181
Beal MC (1967) The subjective factors of palpatory diagnosis. J.O. August: 91–93
Bergsmann O, Eder M (1967) Thorakale Funktionsstörungen. Haug, Heidelberg
Bergsmann O, Eder M (1982) Funktionelle Pathologie und Klinik der Brustwirbelsäule. Bd.2: Funktionelle Pathologie und Klinik der Wirbelsäule. Fischer, Stuttgart New York
Bischoff HP (1983) Segmentale Diagnostik an der Wirbelsäule. Manuelle Medizin heute. Springer, Berlin Heidelberg New York Tokyo, pp 21–27
Bischoff HP (1988) Chirodiagnostische und chirotherapeutische Technik. Perimed, Erlangen
Bittscheid W (1988) Elektromyographische Messungen an der Rückenmuskulatur vor und nach Manipulation. Man Med 26: 47–51
Bourdillon JF, Day EA (1987) Spinal manipulation, 4th edn. William Heinemann Medical Books / Appleton & Lange, London
Bowles CH (1981) Functional technique: A modern perspective. J Am Osteopath Assoc 80: 326–331
Briner B, Conley R, Ward R (1986) Tutorial on level I myofascial release technique. Michigan State University, E. Lansing, Michigan
Brügger A (1977) Die Erkrankungen des Bewegungsapparates und seines Nervensystems. Fischer, Stuttgart New York
Buerger A (1979) Klinische Untersuchungen zur Wirksamkeit der Manuellen Therapie. Theoretische Fortschritte und praktische Erfahrungen der Manuellen Medizin. Konkordia, Bühl, pp 194–213
Corre F le, Rageot E (1979) Über ein klinisches Zeichen bei cervicalen Cephalgien: "Das Zeichen der Augenbraue" nach Maigne. Theoretische Fortschritte und praktische Erfahrungen der Manuellen Medizin. Konkordia, Bühl, pp 68–69
Cyriax J (1969) Textbook of orthopaedic medicine. Bailliére Tindal, London
Dörr WM (1962) Nochmals zu den Menisci in den Wirbelbogengelenken. Z Orthop 96/4: 457
Dvořák J, Dvořák V (1983) Manuelle Medizin Diagnostik. Thieme, Stuttgart New York
Dvořák J, v. Orelli F (1982) The rate of complications in relationship to the number of manipulative procedures performed in Switzerland, Schweiz Rundsch Med Praxis 71: 64
Eder M, Tilscher H (1982) Schmerzsyndrome der Wirbelsäule. Die Wirbelsäule in Forschung und Praxis, vol 81. Hippokrates, Stuttgart
Eder M, Tilscher H (1988) Chirotherapie. Vom Befund zur Behandlung. Hippokrates, Stuttgart
Eklundh M (1979) Achte auf Deinen Rücken! Pflaum, München
Engel JM (1982) Quantitative Thermographie in der Diagnostik und Therapiekontrolle der manuellen Medizin. Man Med 2: 36–43
Erdmann H (1967) Grundzüge einer funktionellen Wirbelsäulenbetrachtung. Man Med 5: 55
Erdmann H (1968a) Grundzüge einer funktionellen Wirbelsäulenbetrachtung. Man Med 6: 32
Erdmann H (1968b) Man Med 6: 78
Fisk JW (1977) The painful neck and back. Thomas, Springfield/Ill
Forte M (1981) Trattato di Medicina Maniplativa. Publ by the Author
Frayette HH (1954) Principles of osteopathic technic. Academy of Applied Osteopathy, Carmel, California

Friberg O (1983) Biomechanics and clinical significance of unrecognized leg length inequality. Paper presented at the International Congress for Manual Medicine, Zurich
Frisch H (1987) Die programmierte Untersuchung des Bewegungsapparats, 2nd edn. Springer, Berlin Heidelberg New York Tokyo
Gaymans F (1973) Neue Mobilisations-Prinzipien und Techniken an der Wirbelsäule. Man Med 2: 12
Gaymans F (1978) Vortrag Internationaler Kongreß für Manuelle Medizin, Kopenhagen
Goodridge JP (1981) Muscle energy technique. Definition, explanation, methods of procedure. J AOA 81: 249
Greenman PE (1979a) Lift therapy: use and abuse. J Am Osteopath Assoc: 238-250
Greenman PE (1979b) Manuelle Therapie am Brustkorb. Man Med 17/2: 17
Greenman PE (1983) Osteopathic update, series 2: layer palpation. Michigan Osteopathic Journal: 36-37
Greenman PE (1984) Eingeschränkte Wirbelbewegung. Man Med 22: 1-15
Greenman PE (1989) Principles of manual medicine. Williams & Wilkins, Baltimore
Grieve GP (1979) Moibilization of the spine, 3rd ed., Churchill Livingstone, Edinburgh
Gutmann G (1968) Das zervikal-diencephal-statische Syndrom des Kleinkindes. Man Med 6: 112-119
Gutmann G (1975a) Röntgendiagnostik der Wirbelsäule unter funktionellen Gesichtspunkten. Man Med 13: 1-12
Gutmann G (1975b) Die pathogenetische Aktualitätsdiagnose. Rehabilitatica 10-11: 15-24
Gutmann G (1982) Funktionelle Pathologie und Klinik der Wirbelsäule. Fischer, Stuttgart New York
Hackett GS (1956) Joint ligament relaxation treated by fibroosseous proliferation. Thomas, Springfield/Ill
Hamberg J, Evjenth O (1982) Muskeldehnung, warum und wie? Remed, Zug
Hansen K, Schliack H (1962) Segmentale Innervation, ihre Bedeutung für Klinik und Praxis. Thieme, Stuttgart
Heilig D (1981) The thrust technique. J Am Osteopath Assoc 81: 244-248
Heufelder D (1983) Zur Beinlängendifferenz. Z Allg Med, pp 440-454
Hildreth AG (1942) The lengthening shadow of Dr. Andrew Taylor Still. Hildreth, Macon, Missouri & Van Vleck, Paw Paw, Michigan
Hoover HV (1958) Functional technique, Yearbook Academy of Applied Osteopathy. Carmel, California
Hülse M, Partsch CJ (1976) Cervicaler Nystagmus ausgelöst durch Halsrezeptoren. HNO 24: 268
Hülse M (1983) Die zervikale Gleichgewichtsstörung. Springer, Berlin Heidelberg New York Tokyo
Huguenin F (1985) Gesunder Rücken. Hallwag, Bern
Janda V (1970) Muskelfunktion in Beziehung zur Entwicklung vertebragener Störungen. Manuelle Medizin und ihre wissenschaftlichen Grundlagen. Verlag für physikalische Medizin, Heidelberg
Janda V (1976) Muskelfunktionsdiagnostik. Steinkopf, Dresden
Jones LH (1981) Strain and counterstrain. Am Acad Osteopathy, Colorado Springs, Colorado
Junghans H (1954) Das Bewegungssegment der Wirbelsäule und seine praktische Bedeutung. Arch Orthop 104
Kaltenborn FM (1976) Manuelle Therapie der Extremitätengelenke. Norlis, Oslo
Kapandji IA (1970) The physiology of joints. Churchill Livingstone, Edinburgh
Kibler M (1958) Das Störungsfeld bei Gelenkerkrankungen und inneren Krankheiten. Hippokrates, Stuttgart
Kimberly PE (1979) Bewegung - Bewegungseinschränkung - Anschlag. Theoretische Fortschritte und praktische Erfahrungen der Manuellen Medizin. Konkordia, Bühl, pp 39-44
Kleynhans AM (1980) Complications of and contraindications to spinal manipulative therapy. In: Haldeman S (ed) Modern developments in the principles and practice of chiropractic. Appleton Century Crofts, New York, pp 359-384
Korr IM (1975) Proprioceptors and somatic dysfunction. JAOA 74: 638
Kuhlendahl H (1970) Analyse der Biomechanik von Halswirbelsäule und Rückenmark. In: Trostdorf E, Steuder HS (eds) Wirbelsäule und Nervensystem. Thieme, Stuttgart
Kunert W (1975) Wirbelsäule und Innere Medizin. Enke, Stuttgart

References

Lanz-Wachsmuth (1982) Praktische Anatomie II, 7 Rücken. Springer, Berlin Heidelberg New York Tokyo
Lewit K (1977) Manuelle Medizin im Rahmen der medizinischen Rehabilitation. Urban & Schwarzenberg, München
Lewit K (1981) Muskelfazilitations- und Inhibitationstechniken in der Manuellen Medizin. Man Med 19/1, 2: 12, 40
Lewit K (1985) Manipulative therapy in rehabilitation of the motor system. Butterworths, London Boston Durban Singapore Sydney Toronto Wellington
Lewit K, Gaymans F (1980) Muskelfazilitations- und Inhibitationstechniken in der Manuellen Medizin. Man Med 18/6: 102
Magoun HJ (1976) Osteopathy in the cranial field. The Journal Printing Co., Kirksville
Maigne R (1961) Die manuelle Wirbelsäulentherapie. In: Die Wirbelsäule in Forschung und Praxis, vol 22. Hippokrates, Stuttgart
Maitland GD (1977) Vertebral Manipulation, 3rd edn. Butterworth, London
Manca S, Niepel G, Dinka I (1977) Anteil der Kokzygodynie an den Kreuzschmerzen. Man Med 15: 32-34
Menell J (1952) The science and art of joint manipulation. In: The spinal column vol II. Churchill, London
Mitchell FL, Prusso NA, Moran PS (1979) An evaluation and treatment manual of osteopathic muscle energy. ICEOP, Valley Park
Neumann H-D (1978) Scriptum zum Informationskurs der Deutschen Gesellschaft für Manuelle Medizin, 2nd edn. Konkordia, Bühl
Neumann H-D (1979) Ein didaktisches Denkmodell zur Manuellen Medizin. Theoretische Fortschritte und praktische Erfahrungen der Manuellen Medizin. Konkordia, Bühl, pp 244-251
Neumann H-D (1980) Diagnosis and treatment of pelvic girdle lesions. In: Greenmann PE (ed) Concepts and mechanisms of neuromuscular functions. Edited by Phil. E. Greenman. Springer, Berlin Heidelberg New York Tokyo
Neumann H-D (1985) Manuelle Diagnostik und Therapie von Blockierungen der Kreuzdarmbeingelenke nach F. Mitchell. Man Med 23: 116-126
Neumann H-D (1988) Die Behandlung der HWS mit der Muskelenergietechnik nach Mitchell. Man Med 26: 17-25
Neumann H-D, Wolff H-D (1979) Theoretische Fortschritte und praktische Erfahrungen der Manuellen Medizin. Konkordia, Bühl
Niethard FU (1982) Formveränderungen der Lendenwirbelsäule bei Beinlängendifferenz. Zschr f Orth u ihre Grenzgeb 120, 2: 91-214
Palmer SG (1933) The subluxation specific – the adjustment specific. Davenpurt, Iowa
Paterson JK, Burn L (1985) An introduction to medical manipulation. MTP Press Limited, Lancaster, Boston, The Hague, Dordrecht
Paterson JK, Burn L (1986) Examination of the Back. MTP Press Limited Lancaster, Boston, The Hague, Dordrecht
Peper W (1978) Der chiropraktische Report. Haug, Heidelberg
Polacek P (1966) Receptors of the joints (their structure, variability and classification) Lekarska fakulta, University J. E. Pukyne, Brunn, Czechoslovakia
Rompe G (1978) Beinlängendifferenzen. Informationen d Berufsverb Orth 2: 31
Sachse J (1977) Manuelle Untersuchung und Mobilisationsbehandlung der Extremitätengelenke. Fischer, Heidelberg (Schriftenreihe Manuelle Medizin, vol 4)
Sachse J (1979) Hypermobilität, Einteilung und diagnostische Kriterien. Theoretische Fortschritte und praktische Erfahrungen der Manuellen Medizin. Konkordia, Bühl, pp 154-158
Sandberg LB (1955) Atlas und Axis. Hippokrates, Stuttgart
Schiötz EH, Cyriax J (1975) Manipulation past and present. Heinemann Medical Books, London
Schmitt HP (1978) Manuelle Therapie der Halswirbelsäule und ihre Gefahren. Man Med 16: 71-77
Schneider W, Tritschler T, Dvořák J, Dvořák V (1984) Ausbildungskonzept Manuelle Medizin in der Schweiz 1983. Man Med 22: 139-144
Schwarz E (1970) Internistische Indikationen der manipulativen Therapie. Man Med 2: 25
Seifert K (1981) Cervical-vertebragene Schluckschmerzen in der HNO-Heilkunde. Man Med 19: 85-91

Seifert K (1988) The functional disturbances of the cervical spinal joints and their role in peripheral, vestibular vertigo. Man Med 26: 89-94
Sell K (1969) Spezielle manuelle Segmenttechnik als Mittel zur Abklärung spondylogener Zusammenhangsfragen. Man Med 7: 2
Spalteholz-Spanner (1966) Handatlas der Anatomie des Menschen. Scheltema & Holkeman, Amsterdam
Steglich H-D (1974) Zur Druckbelastung des Stützgewebes durch manual-therapeutische Techniken. Paper presented at the International Congress of Manual Medicine, Prague
Steinbrück K, Rompe G (1979) Hochleistungssport - planmäßig erworbene Hypermobilität? Theoretische Fortschritte und praktische Erfahrungen der Manuellen Medizin. Konkordia, Bühl, pp 159-164
Steinrücken H (1980) Chirotherapeutisch beeinflußbare Krankheitsbilder. Hippokrates, Stuttgart
Stiles EG (1979) Manuelle Behandlung der chronischen Lungenerkrankungen.Theoretische Fortschritte und praktische Erfahrungen der Manuellen Medizin. Konkordia, Bühl, pp 110-119
Still AT (1908) Autobiography - with a history of the discovery and development of the science of osteopathy. Publ by the Author, Kirksville (Revised edn)
Stoddard A (1961) Manual of Osteopathic Technic. Hutchinson, London
Stoddard A (1982) Leben ohne Rückenschmerzen. Hippokrates, Stuttgart
Sutter M (1975) Klinik und Bedeutung spondylogener Reflexsyndrome. Schweiz Rundsch Med Prax 64: 42
Terrier JC (1969) Die manipulative Therapie der Wirbelsäule: Grundlagen und Indikationen. Rheumatismus in Forschung und Praxis, vol V. Huber, Bern Stuttgart Wien
Tilscher H (1977) Das obere Zervikalsyndrom. Zschr f Orth u ihre Grenzgeb 6: 112
Ward RC, Sprafka S (1981) The Project on Osteopathic Principles, Glossary of osteopathic terminology. J Am Osteopath Assoc 80: 552-567
White A, Panjabi MM (1978) Clinical biomechanics of the spine. Lippincott, Philadelphia
Winkel D et al. (1985) Nicht operative Therapie der Weichteile des Bewegungsapparates, Teil 2. Gustav Fischer, Stuttgart New York
Wolf J (1969) Die Chondrosynovialmembran als einheitliche Auskleidungshaut der Gelenkhöhle mit Gleit- und Barrierefunktion. Man Med II: 25
Wolff H-D (1983) Neurophysiologische Aspekte der Manuellen Medizin. Springer, Berlin Heidelberg New York
Wyke BD (1979) Reflexsysteme in der Brustwirbelsäule. Theoretische Fortschritte und praktische Erfahrungen der Manuellen Medizin. Konkordia, Bühl, pp 99-100
Wyke BD, Polacek (1975) Articular neurology - the present position. J Bone Joint Surg [Br] 57: 401
Zicha K (1966) Rehabilitation der rheumatischen Arthritis. Physikal Med Rehab 7: 261
Zicha K (1979) Proliferationstherapie bei Enthesopathien. Theoretische Fortschritte und praktische Erfahrungen der Manuellen Medizin. Konkordia, Bühl, pp 190-193
Zukschwerdt L, Emminger E, Biedermann F, Zettel H (1960) Wirbelgelenk und Bandscheibe. Hippokrates, Stuttgart

10 Subject Index

Abnormal loading forces 90
Active mobilization 68
Anatomical changes with trauma 78
Anatomical motion barrier 27
Ankylosing spondylitis 79
"ART" 15
Articulatory technique 67
Asymmetry 15

Barrier engagement
   direct 64
   indirect 64
Basic plumb-line 55
Blockage 3
Bone setting 1

Capsular pattern 58
Cardiac disease
   dysrhythmia 93
   ischemia 93
Cardiovascular reflex 9
Carpal tunnel syndrome 91
Cervical syndrome 88
Chiropractic 2
Clinical cases 88 ff.
Close packed position 34
Coccydynia 100
Complications, vertebral artery 81
Contraindications to manual medicine 79
Convex-concave rule 67
Counseling 77
Cranio-sacral technique 76

Degenerative changes 79
De Kleyn hanging test 83
Destructive processes 78
Diagnosis in manual medicine 16
   general 16
   scan 15, 22
   screen 15
   segmental 16
   specific 16
Differential diagnosis, ruptured lumbar disc 98
Dizziness 88

Documentation 37
Downslip 99
Drop attacks 83
Dynamic neutral position 72
Dysrhythmia 93

Empty end-feel 30
End-feel 22, 28
   "empty" 30
   pathological 30
   physiological 30
Epicondylitis
   lateral 91
   medial 91
Exercise regimen 87
Extremity joints
   examination 57
   therapy 100

Facilitation 8
Fast twitch fibers 59, 60
Faulty movement 13
Faulty posture 89
Fryette's rules 32
Functional technique 71
Functional unit 6

Gastrointestinal reflex 9
General hypermobility 85
Gliding mobilization 66

Headache 88, 90
Head plumb-line 55
Hearing difficulties 88
Heel lift 96
Hormonal influences 85
Hypermobility
   general 85
   joint play 86
   localized 86
   X-ray evaluation 86

Identification muscles 11
Impulse force 74
Indicator muscles 11
Indirect techniques 71

Inflammatory processes 78
Inflare 99

Joint end-feel 22
Joint play 30, 58, 86
Joint resiliency 22

Landmarks
   extremities 16
   spine 17, 18
Layer palpation 19
Leg length 45
Length testing, muscles 60
Loading forces 7, 13
Local hypermobility 86
Local segmental irritation 46
   cervical spine 46
   costotransverse joints 50
   lumbar spine 48
   sacro-iliac joint 51
   thoracic spine 48
Low amplitude, high velocity
   technique 73
Lower cervical syndrome 91
Lumbar disc herniation 96
Lumbar syndrome 94

Manipulation 1
Manual medicine
   diagnosis 16
   theoretical model 5
   therapy 62
Manual therapy 62 ff.
Mechanical circuit 6
Metastases 79
Mistakes in muscle energy technique 69
Mobilization
   with impulse (thrust) 73
   without impulse 65
Motion barrier
   anatomical 27
   pathological 27
   physiological 27
Motion testing 38
   cervical spine 38
   lumbar spine 42
   rib joints 42
   sacro-iliac joint 44
   thoracic spine 40
Muscle chains 53
Muscle energy technique 68
Muscular balance 59
Myofascial technique 76

Neutral position 72
Nociceptors 8
Nutation 25
Nystagmus 83

Osteopathy 1
Osteoporosis 80
Outflare 99

Palpable band 11
Palpation 19
Palpatory technique 22
Passive mobilization 65
Pathological hypermobility 86
Pathological motion barrier 27
Pelvic belt 87
Pelvic torsion 45
Peripheral segmental irritation 52
Phasic muscles 59 f.
Physical therapy 63, 87
Physiological motion 32
   barrier 27
Plumb-line
   basic 55
   head 55
Postural muscles 60
Pre-tensing 74
Present neutral position 72
Proliferation therapy 87
Proprioceptors 8
Provisional treatment 88
Provocative testing 10
Pseudo-Lasègue 51, 98
Psychological disturbances 84, 90
Psychotherapy 77

Radiographic findings, normal 56
Radiographic technique 54
Range of motion 15
Record keeping 37
Reevaluation 76
Reflex circuit 7
Reflexes
   cardiovascular 9
   gastrointestinal 9
Rehabilitation 63
Respiratory release technique 71
Restrictive barrier 64
Ruptured lumbar disc 97

Sacro-iliac joint 97
   motion 25
Scan 15, 22
Sciatica 96
Sclerosing therapy 87
Screen 15
Seated flexion test 44
Segmental irritation
   local 11
   peripheral 11
Segmental manual examination 34
Segmental tender points 10
Shoe lift 90

Subject Index

Silent dysfunction 9
Slack 34
Slow twitch fibers 60
SOAP format 15
Soft tissue techniques 64
Somatic dysfunction
   causes 13
   definition 4
   hypotheses 4
   role 13
   significance 13
Somato-visceral reflex 10
Space occupying lesion 90
Specific manual examination 22
Spinal nerve 10
Spinal segment 5
Splinting 87
Standing flexion test 44
Strain-counterstrain technique 73
Strength testing, muscles 60
Sudeck's atrophy 79
Summation 9
Surface orientation 16
Syncope 83

Team approach 63
Technique
   active mobilization 68
   articulatory 67
   cranio-sacral 76
   direct 64
   functional 71
   gliding mobilization 66
   indirect 71
   low amplitude, high velocity (thrust) 73
   mobilization with impulse 73
      without impulse 65
   muscle energy 68
   myofascial 76
   passive mobilization 65
   respiratory release 71
   soft tissue 64
   strain-counterstrain 73
   thrust 73
   traction 66
   visual facilitation 70
Test traction 83
Thoracic syndrome 90
Thrust technique 73
Tissue texture abnormality 15
Tonic muscles 59 f.
Traction 66
Trauma 78
Tumor 79

Upper cervical syndrome 89
Upslip 99

Vertebral artery 81
Vertebral-basilar insufficiency 83
Vertigo 83
Viscero-somatic reflex 10
Visual facilitation technique 70

X-ray examination 53

Zone of irritation 10